A Life in Public Health

An Insider's Retrospective

Lester Breslow received his education at the University of Minnesota, earning his B.A. (1935), M.D. (1938), M.P.H. (1941), and Sc.D. (Hon.) (1988). After two years with the Minnesota Department of Health and then military service with the seventh infantry division in World War II he joined the California Department of Public Health in 1946 to found the Bureau of Chronic Diseases. He left the Department in 1967 after serving as State Health Officer to become a professor at the UCLA School of Public Health, then Chairman of the UCLA Medical School's Department of Preventive and Social Medicine. Thereafter, he served as Dean, UCLA School of Public Health (1972–1980), following which he retired but has continued public health activity to the present time, 2004. Dr. Breslow has been President of the International Epidemiology Association, the American Public Health Association, and the Association of Schools of Public Health; he is a member of the Institute of Medicine. He has received the Lasker Award, Sedgwick Medal of the American Public Health Association, Dana Award, Healthtrac Award, and the Lienhard Award of the Institute of Medicine, National Academy of Sciences.

Dr. Breslow has served as Director of Studies for President Truman's Commission on Health Needs of the Nation, the University of California's Health Plan Grading System, and the National Cancer Institute's report on Cancer Control Objectives for the Nation 1985–2000. He initiated California's chronic disease control program and the Human Population Laboratory including its health studies in Alameda County, and played a leading role in California's tobacco control program. He was the founding editor of the *Annual Review of Public Health* and editor-in-chief of the *Encyclopedia of Public Health*.

A Life in Public Health

An Insider's Retrospective

Lester Breslow, MD, MPH

 Springer Publishing Company

Springer Publishing Company, Inc.
11 West 42nd Street, 15th Floor
New York, NY 10036-8002

Acquisitions Editor: Ursula Springer
Production Editor: Jeanne Libby
Cover design by Joanne Honigman

01 02 03 04 05/5 4 3 2 1

Breslow, Lester.
  A life in public health : an insiders's retrospective / Lester
Breslow.
      p. ; cm.
   Includes bibliographical references and index.
   ISBN 0-8261-2714-2
   1. Breslow, Lester. 2. Public health personnel—United
States—Biography.
      [DNLM: 1. Breslow, Lester. 2. Physicians—United States—
Personal Narratives. 3. Public Health—United States—Personal
Narratives. WZ 100 B8425 2004] I. Title.
RA424.5.B74A3 2004
610'.92—dc22   2004019614

Printed in the United States of America by Maple-Vail Book Manufacturing Group.

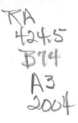

To my wife, Devra,
and to my many colleagues
through the years of a career in public health

Contents

Introduction

I n writing *A Life in Public Health: An Insider's Retrospective,* my aim is to note some of the major public health developments of the latter half of the twentieth century and to describe the principal aspects of my participation in them. The account is intended to indicate how society has coped with important trends in health problems, and how a public health worker can take part in achieving the favorable ones that have characterized recent decades. Some historical background on features of public health is also included, as well as some autobiographical detail.

Tremendous progress in disease control (first against the communicable diseases) has extended longevity from only 47 years in 1900 to 77 years in 2000. During the mid-century years, when noncommunicable, chronic diseases became the dominant health problem, it became clear that public health could not be limited to communicable disease control activities. Advances against those chronic diseases have characterized the second half of the century, and a larger view of necessary public health action has arisen. That has entailed struggles to incorporate chronic disease control and appropriate responsibility for medical care, particularly ensuring access to good quality services, into public health.

The view that public health embraces three types of services—environmental, medical, and behavioral—to improve health has accompanied discoveries that these three fields include both the major determinants of health and the opportunities for progress. The importance of a behavioral approach to health in the current period has emerged from the findings that certain behaviors, e.g., smoking, are predominant factors in the chronic disease epidemic. Reduction of tobacco use has thus become a major public health activity in which California has taken the lead.

In addition to delineating these current aspects of public health, I indicate how public health administration in the United States has evolved to cope with the new health circumstances. A further chapter indicates major features of international health with emphasis on international collaboration in epidemiology and the relationship of developed and developing countries. Reflecting the latter part of my career, I indicate how academic public health fits into the picture with particular attention to my own institution, the UCLA School of Public Health.

In closing I offer some observations and recommendations from a career touching several public health developments during the latter half of the twentieth century. It has provided exhilarating opportunities.

Personal Life 1

I was born in 1915 in Bismarck, North Dakota. When I mention my birthplace people often ask how someone of Eastern European ancestry happened to be born there. The answer is that my father, Joseph Breslow, had gone west to escape New York's Lower East Side where his mother had brought him and his older sister from the "old country." His father had died there in an occupational accident. Living on Hester Street and working as a child in the garment industry, my father hated every aspect of that Jewish ghetto life: the crowded living conditions, the work, the food, and the religion.

Inspired by some chemistry lectures, which he attended at Cooper Union, my father became a pharmacist. As soon as he had earned enough money for the move, he ventured "out west" with his mother and sister and opened a drugstore in Glen Ullin, North Dakota. Being adept at languages Joe also served as general town translator for transactions between local merchants and people in the several ethnic enclaves from Germany and Eastern European countries who had established them-selves in southwestern, rural North Dakota.

Still shunning Jewishness, when the time came for marriage, he never-theless sought a "nice Jewish girl" as a wife. At the suggestion of his local associate, the doctor, he journeyed to Frankfurt, Michigan, to consider the six daughters in the Danziger family. He persuaded the father to let the one my father selected, though not the eldest, go first. After courting and marrying Mayme, who had been an elementary school teacher, he brought her to Bismarck, where he was just moving to start a new drug store, and there they raised a family of three boys of whom I was the eldest. My brothers, Sidney and Arthur, both arrived within three years of my birth, which meant a busy early life for our mother.

In our small-town, middle-class life my father participated fully in the business community while my mother was socially active and highly reputed as an excellent cook. My life as a youngster, fairly typical of growing up in that milieu, included selling *Liberty Magazine* on Fridays and Sunday newspapers from the Twin Cities, as well as delivering prescriptions from my father's drug store to the local hospital. After several years of such work my savings of more than $300 were unfortunately lost when the local bank failed in 1927 as an early casualty of the Great Depression.

From those days in Bismarck I recall the winter cold and sledding down the hard-snowed street near our house, which the police had blocked off to traffic; helping my father shovel coal into our basement furnace; the 25- and 50-pound blocks of ice the iceman left in the refrigerator during the hot summer months; the barbershop for men with the big spittoon at the doorway; the Ku Klux Klan parade going past our house; annual visits by the circus; Saturday afternoons at the movie house watching Tom Mix, the cowboy movie actor who at the end of the show kissed his big white horse, Tony, rather than the heroine; our summer vacations at Lake Melissa in Minnesota; and occasional visits to my mother's family in Columbus, Ohio.

In our family we were conscious of being Jewish but were not observant beyond attending High Holy Day services that were performed by itinerant leaders (not really rabbis) in the second-floor room above our drugstore, and eating matzos during Passover. Although my parents played bridge with some members of the local country club, they were not invited to join that club because in Bismarck at that time being Jewish meant being kept outside definite social boundaries. Although the more orthodox Jewish people isolated themselves socially, my parents went the limit in mingling with the gentiles; they also had good friends among the few Jewish businessmen's families. I was always aware of our separateness but not really bothered by it.

Our home in Bismarck was not characterized by much display of affection. It was a three-brother household with my father usually at the store and at home mainly for meals and my mother busy preparing food, maintaining clothes, and cleaning house. Dad did teach me how to drive the family automobile on the road to Fort Lincoln, a small military post near Bismarck, but offered no other instructions in special skills that I recall. Mother more explicitly enunciated the family expectations: hard work in school and elsewhere, politeness, honesty, and thrift.

When I was 13, the family moved briefly to South St. Paul and then settled in Minneapolis, where our long-awaited sister was born. In Minneapolis my father at first turned away from pharmacy as a way of making a living. His several business ventures during the Depression's first few years took our living standards down considerably below what he had anticipated when leaving Bismarck. Initially he bought and operated a confectionery-ice cream store. When the deepening Depression severely diminished income from that business, he sold it and joined one of my mother's brothers in a taxicab company. Uncle Lou mainly smoked cigars around the office and shouted orders, while my father handled the money, but failure to keep the City Council "properly involved" led that enterprise to a bad end. My father then backed a clever dress-cutter in manufacturing dresses, but he soon forced Dad out of the business, leading to a further loss. Finally, after all these failures he bought a small drug store opposite the Northwestern Hospital, where he worked long hours, alone in the store most days and evenings, in order to keep us afloat through the middle 1930s.

HIGH SCHOOL, COLLEGE, AND MEDICAL SCHOOL

From 1928 to 1932 I attended West High School in Minneapolis, taking the streetcar each morning from the southwest side of Lake Harriet where we lived. My worst childhood experience extended into those high school years from the age of 3 when I had begun suffering from such severe stammering that I never raised my hand in the classroom even when I knew the answer to a teacher's question. I did well in my studies, which included Latin, journalism, geometry, and algebra, but did not participate in school social activities. (Fifty years after graduation I began going to class reunions every five years, the latest being the 65th in 1997. Those occasions in Minneapolis have yielded much joy, although some regret at having missed so much as a teen-ager.) During my high school years I became keenly aware that my mother dominated our household; she was generous, stern, and a strict disciplinarian. My bar mitzvah experience was not too painful, just another thing my mother expected. However, I thoroughly adopted my father's attitude regarding Jewish (or any) religious activities, which were just ritual and without any other meaning for me.

When I was about 16, I recovered from the speech defect with special treatment that involved being maneuvered by my therapist and teachers into the high school DePol (debating and politics) club, an experience that profoundly influenced my life. Belonging to that club I acquired platform ease and learned to speak clearly by talking to audiences rather than to individuals. That is probably why, as associates must still note to their despair, I often speak to small groups and sometimes even to individuals as though I were on a platform.

My first substantial platform appearance consisted of being the high school graduation speaker. I was elected to this position by the students, even though I was not the valedictorian, evidently because of respect for my having overcome the speech defect and being a good student though not receiving "straight A's" like the four girl valedictorians who were not popular themselves. Participating in the DePol Club also enhanced my emerging left-wing sociopolitical views, which had been aroused by a neighbor who introduced me to socialist books, newspapers, and magazines of the early 1930s. Discussions with that early political mentor intrigued me, but the trend in my thinking greatly irritated my father, who opposed all things governmental. My leftist views probably constituted the "adolescent break" from him; and my ideological conversion continued. Other intellectual interests included work on the *West High Weekly*, the school's newspaper, on which I served as editor during my senior year. A significant event in my speech therapy involved reading Clifford Beer's book, *A Mind that Found Itself* (Beers, 1921), a favorite of my speech mentor who wanted to introduce me to larger aspects of mental health to facilitate the therapy. That autobiography of a psychotic man who recovered from his illness stimulated my resolve to help people with mental problems, and led to my becoming a psychiatrist.

A student tour to Europe, a high school graduation present from my parents in the summer of 1932, permitted visits to the usual attractions in London and Paris; however, Munich provided more memorable experiences: my first opera—a magnificent performance of *Figaro's Hochzeit*—and my encounter with the Nazi movement. Some of the American students had brought firecrackers, which they lit and tossed from our hotel window to celebrate the Fourth of July. The explosions attracted both local police and Nazi storm troopers, who spent hours outside our hotel investigating the situation. That summer Hitler was getting close to power over Germany. By that time Socialist leanings had made me a thorough and somewhat sophisticated anti-Fascist, but I noted that the other students seemed simply amused and failed to understand the situation's political aspects. They saw it as a huge joke, whereas I strongly felt its serious portent for Germany's (and the world's) future. The event heightened my sociopolitical sensitivities, defined my personal isolation from most contemporaries, and increased my sense of separateness.

THE UNIVERSITY

To become a psychiatrist, I attended the University of Minnesota, starting in 1932 for a B.A. degree in 1934, and then medical school, which I completed in 1938. Devotion to my studies at the University and working in my father's drug store two evenings a week and one day each weekend left little time for social or any other activities during that period. Association with radical student groups during those years of the Great Depression, however, led to my participation in the 1936 Minneapolis general strike. The strike grew out of the initial Teamsters Union's intensive organization effort, and when the Teamsters did not achieve victory alone, other unions joined the struggle and practically shut the whole city down. Governor Floyd Olson finally called out the Minnesota National Guard, not seeking to break the strike, as was so commonly done by governors in those days, but attempting to control violence in an orderly way. Before the National Guard was called out, however, university students entered the conflict on both sides. I would tour the city late in the evening and into the early morning hours, accompanying Teamsters fighting with clubs against those trying to break the strike. Because that cost some sleep hours, I often had difficulty staying awake during medical school lectures the next day; classmates at our fiftieth medical class reunion in 1988 reminded me how they had struggled to keep me alert during those lectures. We sat in designated seats (in order for the teacher to monitor attendance more easily), and my classmates gave one student behind me the assignment of keeping me awake so the professor would not throw me out of class.

I lived with my family in our southwest Minneapolis home through high school, college, and the first two years of medical school, but when my parents and siblings departed Minneapolis for Sioux Falls, South Dakota, I moved to a rooming house near the University of Minnesota campus. Studies were almost everything for me then; my social life consisted of an occasional evening with a few left-wing student friends.

MY FIRST MARRIAGE

In that radical student group I met Alice Philp, a graduate student who had come to the University from California, and she became my first real girlfriend. After graduating from Stanford, Alice had come to Minnesota, in order to obtain a doctoral degree in psychology. We were both 21 years old when we met, found that we shared views about society, and became well acquainted through mutual participation in student activities during the years of her graduate work in psychology and my medical studies. Our association became a first love for both of us. Joint commitment to making society a better place as well as personal attraction brought us together; our growing struggles against our families also probably facilitated the match. After completing medical school I went to New York for my internship in 1938. We continued our blossoming relationship by correspondence and in 1938, while she was completing her doctoral thesis and I was interning, she joined me in New York. In 1939 we eloped because our families were so different—hers Presbyterian and mine Jewish—and we knew that they would not approve of the marriage. Our fathers never did accept the union. Our mothers made the best of it, although in my case the marriage was kept relatively secret from my mother's family and alienated me from those who knew about my having married a gentile. Only Betsy Danzinger, my grandmother, would inquire about my well-being when speaking with my mother. When my larger family became aware of my marital situation, the alienation continued for some years.

Upon completion of my two-year internship in New York, Alice and I moved back to Minneapolis to start our careers, hers as a psychologist and mine as a public health physician (to which field I had migrated from psychiatry, as described later) in the Minnesota Department of Health. She did not have much opportunity for professional work during the early and mid-1940s because our three sons occupied so much time and energy. We named our first, born in February 1941, Norman Edward after Norman Bethune, a Canadian physician who had joined the anti-imperialist struggle in China, and Edward Barsky, an American physician who had volunteered for the International Brigade in the Spanish Civil War to preserve the democratic republic against the Fascist onslaught. We thus retained our sociopolitical views, but did not carry our previous student activities into our new family and professional lives.

After about a year in Minneapolis the Department transferred me to Rochester where Alice, Norman, and I settled into a comfortable home. Although my work required travel throughout southeastern Minnesota, it permitted returning home almost every evening in time for dinner. Our life was completely irreligious, with not the slightest thought of attending any religious service of any denomination, and our social life was quite limited, largely confined to members of the office staff.

World War II increasingly disrupted our rather idyllic existence in Rochester and eventually took me away from it. Finally deciding to enroll in the anti-Fascist struggle I joined the U.S. Army as a preventive medicine officer. After a few months of military training in that field I was assigned to the San Francisco Port of Embarkation, where it appeared that my responsibility there would last for some time. I therefore brought my young family from Minnesota so that we could continue living together. In San Francisco we became a family of four when our second son, Jack William, was born in March 1944. Though it was wartime and I was involved with the Army, we soon settled into a comfortable, typical, young army officer-family life. For about a year in San Francisco we were housed in Park Merced, the Metropolitan Life Insurance Company housing development. After Jack was born our attention focused on his infancy care as well as Norman's childhood development. Again, fortunately, my work permitted being at home a great deal. My assignment to the Pacific Theater thereafter, however, meant a busy time for Alice, especially when our third son, Stephen, was born while I was still overseas. His birthday, May 12, 1945, coincided with VE (Victory in Europe day), the last day the Army counted children for an additional six points toward discharge. Mine came in late 1945.

Upon my return from the Army, life resumed with my family. At first we still lived in Park Merced and I worked for the California State Department of Health, whose main office was then located in San Francisco. Shortly, however, the Department headquarters and our family moved to Berkeley, where our three boys grew from their preschool years into adolescence.

For about fifteen years we lived a stable family life in Berkeley, focused socially as well as professionally on the Department. Alice, a psychology faculty member, became increasingly absorbed at San Francisco State College, but she did not bring her colleagues into our Berkeley social situation.

During the late 1940s and early 1950s I enjoyed taking my sons camping at sites on our own with sleeping bags and at Boy Scout Camp, which I attended as the camp doctor and thus got them admitted while they were still too young to go as scouts. We enjoyed our many experiences in Scout camp life. On one occasion, though, I was explaining to a group of scouts how to deal with a snake bite, using as a prop a small rattlesnake that someone had captured and placed in a glass jar with a lid. Somehow the lid toppled off while my hand was over the jar and the snake leaped up, barely touching a finger with its fangs but clearly leaving two red spots. It was thus necessary for me to demonstrate the treatment on myself: cutting with a scout knife into the spots that the snake's fangs had created, pressing blood out, and then placing a tourniquet on myself. My sons and the other boys watching the demonstration seemed enraptured, but it was not a pleasant way for me to maintain credibility.

Later I took each son during his adolescence on a trip to Europe, in connection with professional trips there that I extended for personal pleasure with them. In retrospect, my main regret about that period in my life was allowing my intense commitment to professional activities to preclude more pleasurable time with my sons. I had practically no interest in sports, for example, and did little in that regard except for getting them started on tennis.

Although my marriage with Alice had lasted several years as a good one, we gradually became estranged as she devoted increasing time to her San Francisco situation while I focused on department colleagues in Berkeley. Unfortunately, the marriage thus began to fail in the early 1960s. When I had become totally disaffected and had moved out of the house, we did see a psychiatrist as a marriage counselor who allowed us only six visits because he was soon starting a long trip. On the last occasion, and with no progress apparent during the first five sessions, he announced when we arrived at his table, "Today we'll take a vote. I vote for divorce." Turning to Alice, who had been strenuously seeking to maintain the marriage but which I regarded as clearly over, he then asked, "And how do you vote?" After her expected response he then turned to inquire of me, "And you?" That made me suddenly realize that the resolution was up to me, and I finally initiated the legal action that culminated in divorce in 1967.

SECOND MARRIAGE

During this time, on a professional trip one wintry evening in Chicago's O'Hare Airport I reached the ticket counter seeking passage to San Francisco. Told that there were no planes going directly to San Francisco that night, I quickly arranged to go by way of Los Angeles. In line just after me came someone wrapped in a ski suit so bulky one couldn't tell if it was "animal, vegetable or mineral." It turned out to be a young woman who was told flatly, "no planes to San Francisco," and nothing further. Overhearing that conversation outraged me, and I told the man behind the counter to "fix her up the same way you did me." Though somewhat wary of the arrangement she agreed, and I helped carry her bags onto the plane. After we were in the air, I asked her about a drink and she replied, "Canadian whiskey." Noticing her now really for the first time, I thought, "This must be some sophisticated babe." Because the drinks were a dollar each and I had only a one dollar and a twenty dollar bill, which the stewardess (not flight attendant in the mid-1960s) could not change, my companion paid for her own drink.

During our discussion on the plane ride she indicated that she was looking for a University of California position as a report writer. If unsuccessful there, I suggested that she might try the California Department of Public Health, located across the street from the University. Subsequently we did find temporary work for her, and she turned out to be an excellent writer and a very agreeable co-worker. Some months later I rediscovered her, well ensconced in civil service and available for a date. Gradually I learned that Devra offered good and inspiring companionship; she was also an excellent cook and enjoyed many friends. During a multiple-year (I thought "secret,") affair, while I lived alone in Berkeley legally separated from my first wife, Devra and I had come to love one another. We decided to get married as soon as my divorce was final.

By that time, in August 1967, I had met and enjoyed many of her friends. When informed about the matter my family was delighted because, among many other desirable characteristics, she was a "nice Jewish girl." Both families joined extensively in the wedding, which was performed by her uncle, a rabbi. Her spontaneity as well as pleasure in entertaining and travel created a new life for me. After an idyllic honeymoon in the Caribbean, Devra and I journeyed to Yale, New York City, and Los Angeles to explore new job opportunities, and ultimately decided on UCLA. As we left for her house in our second loaded car for the final drive to the Southland, Devra said that we had to stop at Josephs, the Berkeley liquor store. Asked why, she said that she had bought a case of wine. When I expressed wonderment that we had to take that purchase for the trip, she quite seriously replied, "I'm not sure that we can find wine in Los Angeles." That, of course, reflected a common view then among northern Californians. In our move to Los Angeles Devra at first sorely missed her Bay Area friends, but we made visits there several times a year and Devra began rapidly acquiring many new friends for us in Los Angeles.

I became completely realigned with my mother's relatives as well as with my own brothers and sister and members of Devra's family. My father had died and my mother lived only nineteen months after our marriage, but she did visit us for three weeks in 1968 and we relished that opportunity to be with her.

THE LARGER FAMILY

All of my sons and daughters-in-law (first Gayle Bramwell Breslow, who married Norman), soon came to know and appreciate Devra and our devotion to one another. Norman and Gayle's family, living in Seattle, expanded with the birth of Lauren Louise in 1968 and then Sara in 1972. Meanwhile my youngest son, Steve, married Kathy van Spankeren and their union produced our grandson, Paul. My son Jack remained at the Berkeley home, taking care of his mother. Devra has embraced all my family as her own and maintains communication with them more fully than I do. My own greatest personal delight has been watching my sons' families grow; to know the three grandchildren, and now the great-grandchildren, Benjamin and Ayelet, whom Lauren and her Israeli husband, Ezra, have brought into the world. Fortunately they are all doing well and scores of my favorite stories, illustrated by Devra's photographs, concern them.

In Los Angeles Devra has become the core of my entire family, made my long-time friends her own, and developed numerous new local friends, in addition to maintaining our home and keeping up with her relatives and friends in the Bay area and elsewhere. Only ten minutes from UCLA, where I work, our home has provided great pleasure as a quiet refuge for us, for welcoming relatives, and also for seeing friends from both the neighborhood and work, from elsewhere in Los Angeles, and from other parts of the country and the world. Our foreign guests have brought special delight. When they greet me, now it's usually not with "Hi Les, how are you?" but "Hi Les, how's Devra?"

Devra has enjoyed several careers in Los Angeles. The first was serving as assistant to Founding Dean Mitchell Spellman for six years as he was developing the Drew Medical School in South Los Angeles. Subsequently she initiated an Art That Heals program, mainly with volunteers, for the UCLA Medical Center, at first for cancer patients and then for the general hospital patients. In due course Devra sought to turn her photography skill into remunerative employment. While it hasn't brought much income, it has resulted in several exhibits and much pleasure for others as well as us. Along the way she has assembled a considerable art collection, especially ceramics and glass, and taken many other responsibilities such as assisting Roger Detels, my colleague at UCLA, in organizing the 1990 Los Angeles meeting of the International Epidemiological Association.

From my experience I would say that the greatest treasure a man can have is a wife like Devra.

During the years in Los Angeles, I have also cultivated a hobby; "cultivated" is the right word because it is gardening. I started one weekend when a long-time friend of Devra's was visiting us for the weekend, and Saturday morning she wanted to walk. Explaining that our neighborhood's lack of sidewalks made walking there inconvenient I suggested an alternative: helping me dig rocks out of some hillside space behind our house so that I could then plateau it into a garden. She pitched in vigorously to give me a big boost. It has now developed into a fenced area (to keep out the deer from the adjacent woods) with orange, lemon, plum, peach, fig and apricot trees, and about 400 square feet for vegetables and herbs. They all do reasonably well, though some years, of course, are better than others. It provides opportunity for a weekly two or three hour stint of physical labor and bringing down some things to eat year-round.

Fortunately my health has remained good except for a myocardial infarction when I was nearly 83, an attack that came one morning while I was making coffee. Devra wisely insisted on calling 911 and then a neighbor physician rather than driving me to the hospital herself as I proposed. The ambulance emergency crew, the physician at the hospital who promptly performed an angioplasty and placed a stent in the main coronary artery, and the cardiologist who has cared for me since the episode have, I believe, given me (to the present time) more than six extra years of life for which I am deeply grateful. That time has provided opportunity for many professional as well as personal adventures, and I keep enjoying them. People sometimes ask why, if I'm so smart about health, I had a heart attack. My explanation is that earlier in my life we didn't know all the things that now permit us to minimize the risk of such an event.

Preparation and Start in Public Health 2

FIRST AIM: PSYCHIATRY

My interest in a health career—at first in mental, specifically behavioral, health—had originated during my recovery from stammering. The agony of contemplating speaking, even before actually trying to speak, swept over me several times every day during childhood and early adolescence. It was awful. The private teacher who helped me overcome the disorder incorporated some mental health readings (like the Beers book already mentioned) and career discussions into the treatment, which inspired me to help others with mental disorders. The euphoria that came with being able to speak easily, and particularly being selected by peers for the class address from the high school graduation platform, reinforced the determination to help others with mental disorders.

At age 17, in the fall of 1932 I entered the University of Minnesota to become a psychiatrist. That meant committing myself to an 8–10-year academic program embracing premedical studies, completion of medical school, and special clinical training in psychiatry. Only two years of prescribed college studies were required in those days for admission to medical school, although authorities preferred that students complete their bachelor degrees before seeking entrance. In my case conserving both time and money by allowing only two years for premedical studies were high priorities because it was essential to me to get off family support within the shortest possible time. Besides, I was impatient to start my career.

Those personal decisions were carried out while Americans were experiencing the depths of economic depression. Unemployment rose to peak levels, and inadequate welfare programs left one-third of the nation

13

"ill-fed, ill-clad and ill-housed," as President Franklin Roosevelt expressed it. The situation strengthened my view that our economic system should be drastically changed.

Being at the University during the tumultuous early and middle 1930s afforded me some refuge from the events that were sweeping the country. The world situation produced student radicalism, which attracted me, but at universities in the 1930s left-wing political activity was generally limited to a small section of the student body; most students' sociopolitical views reflected their middle- or upper-class family origins.

Besides the very demanding premedical courses essential for admission to medical school, I also completed college degree work for a major in psychology, intended to augment preparation to become a psychiatrist. Professor of Psychology, Edna Heidbreder, served as my undergraduate advisor. Her text, *Seven Psychologies* (Heidbreder, 1933), opened my eyes to that field's breadth and divergent approaches, although none of the chapters seemed very pertinent to serious mental illness, which I wanted to understand and treat.

The heavy academic load, especially in addition to working in my father's drug store, left no time for social activities or for sports (which did not interest me anyway). Famed football coach Bernie Bierman trained the Minnesota Golden Gophers to win several Big Ten championships during those days. Although Twin City as well as campus excitement filled the fall days, I did not participate and don't recall attending a single game. Absence from such events increased my continuing sense of general social isolation. What little non-study time was available I devoted mainly to left-wing student political activities.

The first two years of the medical school curriculum consisted almost completely of basic medical sciences, including various aspects of anatomy, physiology, bacteriology, and organic chemistry. Physiology was intriguing in that it revealed how the body worked, but none of the other subjects held any substantial interest for me and I endured them only in order to become a psychiatrist.

One feature of the first two medical school years, however, still comes vividly to mind. Moses Barron, an internal medicine practitioner in Minneapolis, would come to the University Hospital as a clinical instructor, and at 8 A.M. on Friday mornings he would meet for the first time, and then examine, a patient in front of the entire freshman class. The interns would have looked through the roster of hospitalized patients in order to select what they regarded as the most difficult diagnostic case. Dr. Barron would demonstrate how to take a history, do a brief physical examination, and then discuss the diagnosis. One morning the patient was described as an unmarried, 51-year-old, white female who was complaining about an abdominal tumor. Dr. Barron examined her and came to the correct diagnosis: pregnancy. That greatly surprised many of us who had thought pregnancy impossible for a woman of such an age. Moreover, in the course of his examination he pulled down the lower eyelids, inspected the conjunctivae, and announced that the hemoglobin level was 51 percent. Turning to the intern standing with the chart, he asked what the laboratory had found. The intern thumbed through the chart and responded that the laboratory report showed 53 percent hemoglobin, whereupon Dr. Barron informed us that one always had to allow 2 percent for laboratory error. From that remark and the class response to it I learned both the value and the humor that can be inherent in clinical judgment. Only later did the significant difference between so-called evidence-based judgment and the all-too-common opinionated medical arrogance become apparent to me.

At that time most physicians in the community were general practitioners who had received their training before the specialty movement took over medical education in the United States, and medical practice thereafter. Individual fee-for-service payment constituted the almost universal mode of compensating physicians. They tended to practice alone, although some substantial groups such as the famed Mayo Clinic in Rochester, Minnesota, had developed and were beginning to popularize the notion that the best medical service could be obtained where groups of physicians expert in the several evolving branches of medicine had assembled and practiced together.

Prepayment for group practice medical care was espoused by some and occasionally even implemented, as in the Los Angeles Ross-Loos Clinic and the Elk City, Oklahoma, Farmers Union Cooperative Hospital Association (Sinai, Anderson, & Dollar, 1946). As the Great Depression deepened, forward-thinking physicians led both these efforts to ensure medical services for people with low incomes. Organized medicine, however, bitterly opposed such group practice prepayment arrangements as well as government-sponsored health insurance, which by that time prevailed in many countries. President Roosevelt apparently had wanted to include health insurance in his Social Security program to combat the Depression's economic and social effects, but the American Medical Association had fought so strongly and effectively against the notion that Roosevelt dropped it, fearing that including it in the legislation might scuttle the entire program.

In addition to the heavy, basic medical science studies, I acquired some experience while waiting on customers at my father's drugstore evenings and weekends. For example, we sold Lydia Pinkham's compound and other similar medicines over the counter. Elderly ladies would buy these "tonics," which included a considerable alcoholic content, and take two or three tablespoonfuls before retiring to aid sleep. Buttressed by my growing medical wisdom (which probably never rises higher in one's own mind than during the second medical school year), I succeeded one evening in dissuading an older woman from buying such an item. My ethics, however, were evidently incompatible with the drugstore business of that time. Having witnessed the episode, Dad took me to the door and pointed to the woman leaving our store and hastening to the drugstore across the street, where she apparently made the purchase. So much for that kind of patient education, he explained.

During the summer of 1936, after my second year in medical school, I decided that the time had arrived to start specific studies for psychiatry. In those days this meant neuropsychiatry, so I undertook special laboratory work in neuroanatomy and neuropathology as one basis for entering the field. Examining brain and other neural tissues microscopically thus occupied my summer months following basic science training in medical school. In those days, of course, knowledge of how the brain worked and the corresponding relationships between the anatomic and the behavioral characteristics of life were primitive. The last two medical school years were devoted to clinical training and proved somewhat more interesting than the basic science courses, but I still did not achieve a very good academic record.

During the summer after my third medical school year I sought clinical psychiatric experience at the Fergus Falls State Hospital for the Insane with its 2,200 patients. My duties there consisted of making rounds each morning with one of the four physicians, each of whom saw on the average more than 100 patients daily, mainly on a walk through the wards. While on these rounds I would receive the "call," a telephone summons to assist in the only treatment available in the institution beyond custodial care, namely, insulin shock therapy. The call came about 9:30 each morning when the patients who had been receiving increasing doses of insulin for several days would finally succumb to insulin shock. I would rush over to put gastric tubes down the gullets of those patients who were having convulsions induced by the low blood sugar levels that their insulin injections caused. Pouring sugar solution into their stomachs would bring them out of shock. I did not see any improvement with that therapy during the summer of 1937 and became totally disillusioned with psychiatry as it could be practiced then, i.e., before the recent advances in therapy.

SWITCH TO PUBLIC HEALTH

It became overwhelmingly clear to me that essentially nothing could be done at that time for severely mentally ill patients except keeping them from hurting themselves or others. That summer was a totally disheartening experience, causing me to abandon any thought of psychiatry. Upon my return to medical school that fall, utterly discouraged in my career choice, I was persuaded by a friend that my ideology as a political activist for disadvantaged people better suited me for public health. I then became acquainted with Gaylord Anderson, Minnesota's new professor of public health, and under his tutelage switched to that field in my senior medical school year.

After medical school graduation I obtained internship training at the U.S. Public Health Service Marine Hospital, in Staten Island, New York, hoping to enter the U.S. Public Health Service Corps to pursue a career. During the little time available apart from intensive hospital duties my main social contacts consisted of left-wing medical students and interns in Manhattan, several of whom became lifelong friends. After the second year of internship and my rejection by the Public Health Service as a Corps Officer, I presume because of my political orientation, I returned to Minneapolis where Gaylord Anderson, then Dean of the nascent Minnesota School of Public Health, admitted me to the School. I had also sought admission to Johns Hopkins in order to study with Henry Sigerist, the great scholar of medical history and social medicine, but a favorable decision there came only after I had already started in Minnesota. When I expressed my inclination to accept the late Hopkins offer to Ruth Boynton, Director of the Minnesota Student Health Service where I was temporarily working, she delivered such a stern lecture about the consequences of breaking commitments that I decided to stay in Minnesota.

Immediately after obtaining my MPH degree in 1941 (and also with my medical training) I joined the Minnesota Department of Public Health, where my initial assignment was to become an epidemiologist. Communicable diseases dominated the public health scene everywhere at the time. Smallpox cases still numbered more than a thousand each year in the nation; measles, scarlet fever, and diphtheria affected thousands more. Tuberculosis resulted in well over 50,000 fatalities annually. Although cholera had essentially been eliminated from the United States, malaria still prevailed in the southeastern states. Maternal and child health had sharply improved after Congress passed the Sheppard-Towner

Infant and Maternity Act in 1921, which provided funds for a public health approach to the problem. In the public health world we were oblivious then to the fact that coronary heart disease was rising to prominence and that lung cancer had doubled in the 1930s.

Public health agencies had adopted three types of measures to stop the impact of disease-causing micro-organisms: (1) quarantining infected persons, either in their homes or in special infectious-disease hospitals, (2) preventing the transmission of germs through water and food, and (3) inducing immunity, at first by antitoxins for temporary passive protection of patients after infection had occurred, and later by vaccination of noninfected persons to stop the organisms from establishing themselves and creating an infection. Public health professionals recognized their virtual helplessness against measles, whooping cough, and chicken pox, which were then regarded as essentially inevitable diseases of childhood because they spread person-to-person before isolation could even be attempted, and there were no immunizing agents.

My first experience in the State Department of Public Health was to investigate a small outbreak of typhoid fever in rural Minnesota and trace it to a neighborhood party. Other responsibilities included following up newly diagnosed tuberculosis cases to assure examination of family and other contacts, isolating the patients if their sputum contained tubercle bacilli, and, if necessary, escorting the patients to the sanatorium. Work as an epidemiologist in those days consisted mainly of tracing the chain of infection.

EXPERIENCES AS A LOCAL HEALTH OFFICER

After my first few months of orientation and activity in the Department, Albert Chesley, the State Health Officer, proposed that I go to Rochester (home of the famed Mayo Clinic) to become the District Health Officer for the six southeastern Minnesota counties. Chesley's strategy at that time was to establish such district offices of the State Department of Public Health to assist whatever local personnel were available for public health functions, and to deliver technical services as necessary.

Following Haven Emerson's lead, the American Public Health Association had stipulated six basic local health department activities: vital statistics; sanitation; control of communicable and preventable diseases; laboratory service; protection of health in maternity, infancy, and childhood; and public health education.

It was generally accepted that only jurisdictions including at least 50,000 people could effectively conduct these activities. Municipal health departments, which New York and other large cities had established, were far advanced in organized public health work compared to rural Minnesota. Chesley believed that state district offices would be more effective in the latter situation than local health departments in each small county.

I accepted Chesley's offer and settled with my wife and our son in Rochester, where we lived in a comfortable house within walking distance of my office.

It was exhilarating to feel responsible for public health in that southeastern corner of Minnesota, especially with the previous District Health Officer who had become the Rochester City Health Officer, Floyd Feldman, as my local mentor. Our District staff consisted of a public health nurse who provided consultation (really supervision) to the several visiting nurses employed by various local agencies, and promoted such services where they did not exist; a sanitary engineer who offered technical aid to the several water supply personnel, pasteurization plant operators, and the like; an office administration assistant; and the Health Officer. Aside from learning about public health practice from my District office colleagues, whose activities I was presumably directing, I devoted most of my attention to working with local physicians on communicable disease and maternal and child health problems; personally carrying out epidemiological investigations; and dealing with tuberculosis. Those early experiences evoked in me a very positive attitude toward practicing physicians, most of whom in my Rochester days practiced general medicine rather than the specialties that have become so dominant in more recent times. Only later did that positive attitude become undermined by encounters with some political leaders of what seemed to be a guild-like medical profession that was primarily concerned with its own interests and not supportive of public health. This propensity appeared to expand over the decades, often obstructing public health efforts aimed at improving and extending medical services. In more recent years I have sensed somewhat of a public health–organized medicine rapprochement.

Local public health activity in the early 1940s can be illustrated by the following experience. I recall one morning when the physician in Kasson, a small town located a few miles west of Rochester, called to report that within a few days several dozen children from one school had experienced quite severe flu-like symptoms. I immediately visited his practice and the school, and, assisted by our supervising public health nurse, the sanitary engineer, and some local nurses, I took case histories of the affected youngsters. We also obtained acute and convalescent sera: that is, some blood taken before possible development of immunity, and again after a couple of weeks when immunity would have become established and detectable in the blood. The State Department of Health laboratory, however, could not find an immune response indicating any known pathogenic entity.

Because pigeons frequented the school's roof and thinking that the disease might be some form of psittacosis (parrot fever), we sought some live pigeons at the school so that we could determine whether their blood contained signs of that infection. To obtain the pigeons, my colleagues, Paul Kingston, the District sanitary engineer; Floyd Feldman; and I built a pigeon trap in Feldman's basement. We were well supported by appropriate libations, which his wife provided. Only when we started to carry our contraption up the stairs did we realize that it was too big to move out of the basement. That required taking the cage out in pieces during another long evening and reconstructing it. We then moved the cage to the Kasson school roof and kept it well supplied with bait. Each day we inspected the trap but found no pigeons. On one such occasion, though, as we left the school we encountered a man who asked what we were doing on the roof. When we explained our venture, he asked how many pigeons we wanted. To our reply, "Oh, about a dozen," he responded, "Well, just come over tomorrow morning and I'll have them for you." "We need them alive," I said. "I know," he answered. Somewhat mystified we returned the next morning and were astonished when the man handed us three gunny sacks filled with flopping, very much alive pigeons. To our query as to how he had caught them he explained simply, "I just climbed onto the roof last night with a flashlight. You just shine the light directly into the pigeons' eyes as they're perched there. It seems to paralyze them. Then you pick them off the perch, and put them in the gunny sack." That taught me the importance of finding an expert when you want something unusual done.

Examining the pigeons unfortunately did not reveal the infection's source. Only some years later Monroe Eaton, who directed the virus laboratory in the California State Department of Public Health, reported isolating the agent for what was then called atypical pneumonia, now mycoplasma pneumoniae. Upon testing pairs of acute and convalescent sera from the Kasson epidemic cases, which had been frozen and kept in Minnesota, Eaton found that the sera from the Kasson youngsters showed a very high rise in titer against the virus he had isolated. That led to the second publication of my public health career, a report of an acute respiratory disease outbreak years earlier due to the newly isolated agent. My first paper, published in 1943, had resulted from a study I had started with Gaylord Anderson while I was a student in the School of Public Health. It concerned parental and familial factors in acceptance of diphtheria and smallpox immunization. Those early publications growing directly out of public health practice encouraged me to continue submitting papers on experiences and findings in professional public health work.

By the fall of 1941, as the war spread over Europe, it was increasingly evident that the United States would send soldiers to support our western European allies; Roosevelt was clearly leading the country in that direction. The Japanese Pearl Harbor attack on December 7, 1941, galvanized national action and finally made anti-Fascism thoroughly acceptable. Suddenly our country seemed largely united with that growing effort worldwide.

One morning in Rochester, shortly after our entry into World War II, we received a report that several soldiers at a Wisconsin military training camp just a few miles east of the Minnesota border had contracted syphilis, presumably in a brothel at Winona, Minnesota, a small Mississippi River city in our district. One thing a public health officer cannot tolerate is learning that an infectious disease affecting people in another community originated in his own jurisdiction. That strong feeling impelled me to investigate the epidemic promptly and vigorously. After confirming that the syphilis outbreak was indeed arising from a brothel, which the family of a rather prominent Southeastern Minnesota state senator had allegedly owned for some decades, I sought help from the venereal disease control officer in the headquarters of the Minnesota Department of Public Health. He persuaded Governor Harold Stassen that drastic action must be taken to protect our soldiers. Actually, we had long looked for an opportunity to close the place. At midnight on the Saturday between Christmas and New Year's Day in 1942, a convoy of State police officers arrived from St. Paul in Winona. En route to the house of prostitution they picked up a few local police officers so as to avoid any local tip-off but still not embarrass the local police. The chief social worker from the State Health Department headquarters and I accompanied the raiders. The men were allowed to run away, many holding their trousers and shoes in their hands, while the women were taken to jail. This contrasting treatment illustrated the male chauvinism that has long dominated our approach to prostitution. Monday morning in court the brothel owners faced the penalty that was on the books but had not previously been enforced in Minnesota: any house being operated for prostitution must be padlocked for one year. No use could be made of it; not even entry was allowed. The house owners protested that they knew nothing about what was going on, and that if anything bad was underway it must be the fault of those "bad women." Their argument did not prevail, and the Winona establishment was in fact padlocked for one year.

Comfortable though I had become in Rochester, my strong anti-Fascist feelings prevailed and I felt compelled to volunteer for the Army, though exempted from the draft by virtue of being in public health as well as by having a young child. My sense of guilt for not having joined the anti-Fascist struggle during the Spanish Civil War also entered into my feelings. World War II thus disrupted our almost idyllic existence in Rochester and ultimately led me to join the Army where I became a preventive medicine officer.

Military Life 3

My life in the military began rather inauspiciously. At land grant colleges like the University of Minnesota, all male students at the time were required to participate in the Reserve Officer Training Corps (ROTC). The training offered very little didactic education and nothing about weaponry; I never fired a gun there. Instruction was apparently aimed at indoctrinating male college students to obey military authority, follow orders, and keep pace with others. For most of my contemporaries the ROTC commitment seemed a reasonable requirement for attending a state-supported university, but a few of us strongly opposed the intrusion of militarism into our student days. We hence sought to stop compulsory ROTC.

Involvement with left-wing political groups on the campus led to my becoming leader of a strike against the ROTC at the end of the school year in the spring of 1934. That activity unfortunately made my mother nearly frantic. As I was her eldest son (and the eldest grandson of her parents), she and the whole family had been counting on my admission to medical school and becoming a physician. She felt strongly that my activities were menacing not only my own career but the entire family expectation. The strike did take place during the time that medical school admission decisions were being made, and my mother and I were both conscious of the fact that in those days not many Jewish applicants were allowed to enter. I was terribly sorry to see her suffer so much but believed that my actions justified whatever the consequences might be. That year the medical school dean, Elias Lyon, decided to break the pattern with respect to limiting Jewish student enrollment. Hence, in the entering class of 100 University of Minnesota Medical School students that fall in 1934 several of us were Jewish.

A few of us absented ourselves from the annual spring military parade and instead barricaded ourselves in a second-floor front room of the University Student Union. Standing at that room's large window we spoke in ROTC uniform to about a thousand students gathered below. As evidenced by later disclosure of secret documents showing the U.S. government's involvement, our action, aimed at getting "the Marines out of Nicaragua," did not stop U.S. military support of the corrupt Nicaraguan governments that participated in the exploitation of their people by American interests. Our demonstration against the ROTC, however, probably did serve to bolster enthusiasm among those of us opposed to growing reactionary forces in Europe and their counterparts in the U.S. Against these growing Fascist trends President Roosevelt ultimately became, with Churchill as his close associate, the principal leader of the world's democratic forces.

The Spanish Civil War had strongly highlighted for me what was happening world-wide in the 1930s, when Franco fought with considerable Fascist support from outside Spain to overturn that nation's republican government. When Fascism represented such an obvious threat to peace and security for so many countries, forces from several countries were mobilized to combat it. Americans and others joined an International Brigade to aid the Republic. Though sorely tempted to enlist in that body I did not do so, justifying my inaction by thinking that finishing medical school would be more useful to mankind. Later I felt regret about that decision, especially when I came to know Archie Cochrane, the British epidemiologist best known as founder of the "clinical trial," and others who did volunteer (Bosch, 2003).

ENLISTMENT IN THE ARMY AND FIRST ASSIGNMENTS

The December 7, 1941, bombardment of Pearl Harbor finally catapulted our nation into the war. Though my wife, young son, and I were securely ensconced at that time in Rochester, the World War II Fascist advances were steadily intruding into our social circumstances. Europe was rapidly coming under Nazi control and the Japanese forces were overrunning East Asian and Pacific areas. Although protected from being drafted into military service professionally by being engaged in public health service and personally by having a wife and child, I finally joined the anti-Fascist war. The thought of a world dominated by Hitler, Mussolini, and Hirohito became intolerable to me, and their early victories made that outcome seem quite possible.

In 1943 I volunteered for the U.S. Army Medical Corps. My first assignment took me for training in tropical medicine to the Bethesda Naval Hospital, and the two months there constituted the most rigorous study period of my life. Dedication to the war effort, combined with the learning opportunity, kept me working long hours, but at last my professional public health and political interests coalesced. Enlisting also somewhat assuaged the guilt I felt for not having joined the Spanish republic's anti-Fascist struggle of the late 1930s.

My training continued with field experience in malaria control. For that purpose a few Medical Corps officers were assigned to a field exercise during which we were housed at the Florida State College for Women in Tallahassee, Florida. GIs standing outside but not allowed to enter the compound yelled vulgarities at us as we returned to the campus each evening. We learned primarily by using dynamite to drain swamps where malaria-carrying mosquitoes were breeding, the common practice of engineers who had earlier pursued that approach to preventing malaria in the southeastern United States. A dynamite expert cautioned us that even shaking the dust around sticks of dynamite could result in explosion, and cartons of the stuff should therefore be handled very carefully and never dropped. To illustrate the danger he showed us pictures of men who had been blasted against nearby cement walls because they mishandled dynamite. Seeing those men appear as shadows stuck to the wall deeply impressed us. On the field trip to practice the ditch-draining we young medical officers lined up to lift cases of dynamite from a truck, and then carry them to the swamp site. When my turn came I stepped to the back of the truck like the others and picked up a case. Nobody, however, had made clear to me that dynamite is very heavy. The sudden, unexpected weight on my outstretched arms caused me to drop the case onto my feet. Although the dynamite did not explode, I sensed that my fellow trainees avoided me thereafter.

After tropical medicine training I was assigned as preventive medicine officer to the San Francisco Port of Embarkation, where my principal duty was to assure that no communicable disease problems were brought into port. That entailed my going out about five o'clock A.M. several times a week into the fog covering the San Francisco Bay in a small boat that would carry a few boarding officers to a troop ship that carried mostly returning wounded soldiers, and was en route to dock. After climbing up the rope ladder dangling over the side of the moving vessel I would seek out the medical officer and carry out prescribed formalities for release of the ship from quarantine. The routine consisted mainly of having a cup of coffee with a fellow medical officer on the ship and exchanging some signatures and papers.

On one occasion, however, the visit was more than routine. The ship's medical officer told me that several returning soldiers had died of a suffocating throat disorder during the voyage. Upon investigation it quickly became evident to me that the men had died of throat diphtheria. The disease had spread to returning soldiers during the journey home in the ship's crowded conditions, evidently originating from several patients in the ship's hospital with severe skin diphtheria that they had acquired in the South Pacific. The young medical officers on board the troop ship had not previously seen, and unfortunately did not recognize, throat diphtheria. The causative organisms will grow in wounds under conditions that prevailed in the World War II Pacific Theater, and a substantial number of the returning wounded suffered skin diphtheria. From the latter cases diphtheria bacilli would infect other soldiers on the troop ship, thus yielding the classical, throat form of the disease whose fatal effects could have been avoided by detecting the cases early and giving antitoxin to the patients.

Seeing those dead soldiers stunned me because such deaths were even then nearly always preventable. Knowing that Dr. Karl F. Meyer, Director of the Hooper Foundation at the University of California at San Francisco and a world authority on communicable diseases, was an influential consultant to the Army, I brought the information directly to him. That seemed to me likely to be more effective than going through Army channels. Dr. Meyer invited me to join him for lunch a couple of days later at the San Francisco Family Club. I encountered a highly impressive array of high Army and Navy brass at that luncheon table. After a nice meal, Dr. Meyer, who had placed me at his right hand, asked me to recount the ship-diphtheria story, after which I proposed assuring that adequate stocks of diphtheria antitoxin be placed immediately on board all troop ships, radioing all medical officers with returning troops concerning the diphtheria danger, and instructing all others who might have similar future responsibilities about the matter. Powerful personality that he was, Dr. Meyer then swept the luncheon table group with his hand to emphasize his words, "The lieutenant has described the situation and made his recommendations; now you gentlemen will do what the lieutenant says." The gentlemen appeared a bit discomfited but not inclined to defy Dr. Meyer.

That experience indicated how much the right personal leverage can influence a critical situation. Subsequent events in both civilian and military life reinforced my belief that certain situations justify finding a short-cut way to influence decision makers rather than following bureaucratic channels. Indoctrinating people too strongly in routine officialism often precludes effective action in public health as well as in other circumstances.

PREVENTIVE MEDICAL OFFICER IN THE
SEVENTH INFANTRY DIVISION ON LEYTE

While I was stationed at the San Francisco Port of Embarkation early in 1945, orders came for me to join the Army's Seventh Infantry Division which was then battling for Leyte in the Philippines. Having successfully made the attack on Attu in the Aleutians and then on Kwajelein in the mid-Pacific, the Seventh Division had been selected for that task. Later, examining my route on a C-47 plane to Leyte via Hawaii and Kwajelein to join the Division, I gave profound thanks for that airplane crew's navigational and piloting competence. Arriving one evening with no knowledge of the Seventh Division, completely ignorant of combat, and with no training for it, I reported to Division headquarters carrying orders to be the preventive medicine officer.

My introduction to the situation came the first night when I stood up to urinate. Whispered, colorful expletives from my new comrades promptly taught me where I was and what not to do. Especially at nighttime, never do anything that might attract attention to one's location because doing so might invite Japanese sniper fire. Urinate immediately before you lie down for the night, and if you can't wait till the morning, just roll over a few feet. Indoctrination into battle culture continued with learning how to bathe with water in a helmet, and how to wash one's clothes in a river.

The Headquarters staff did not know what a preventive medical officer should do, and I wasn't too sure myself. As a physician, however, my first point during the intense battle was to ascertain how I could help care for the heavy casualties that were flowing into the clearing station, a quasi-hospital for the Division's approximately 15,000 soldiers. Our situation was akin to that depicted in the TV *MASH* program—except that our unit included no female nurses. Having essentially no competence in the surgical treatment of battle trauma, as my new medical colleagues disappointedly but immediately confirmed, I was assigned to the "shock tent." There we received the severely wounded soldiers who needed blood transfusions and other preliminary treatment. We cared for the worst cases, mostly those with bloody, dirty, penetrating wounds, aiming to keep the soldiers alive a few hours until the surgeons could provide further treatment.

My preventive medicine role on Leyte began when we encountered an epidemic of schistosomiasis. Noting that several soldiers from the Division's engineer battalion reported suffering severely from chills, severe headache, fever, and often dermatitis, I suspected schistosomiasis because the engineers had been building bridges across slow streams, and that work necessitated their spending hours in the river water where they had possibly been exposed to the causative agents. These agents pass one stage of their life cycle in snails that flourish in shallow, slow-moving water, and then escape to bore into a passing human's skin and proceed to the intestine and liver, where they cause extensive pathology. Human (or animal) excrement then reinfects the water where the snails pick up the organisms again. Though schistosomiasis occurs on several continents and islands, a particularly virulent form (*S. japonicum*) prevails in the Southeast Asian areas. The tropical medicine training course had emphasized the condition, and I had been on the lookout for it.

Examining the patients' blood smears with a microscope I found a very high eosinophilia rate. This type of white blood cell increases sharply in parasitic infections such as schistosomiasis. Observing the typical symptoms, ascertaining the eosinophilia count, and noting that the disease outbreak affected only men who had been exposed to slow-moving water made it easy to conclude that we were dealing with schistosomiasis. It attacked several dozen men in that engineer's battalion for whom I recommended evacuation because their illness would continue for several weeks. That was hardly complete preventive medicine, but at least it was recognition of a disease exotic to American medical officers.

After firm military control of Leyte was established, the Division's Special Services Officer introduced the drinking routine at Headquarters. There was, of course, no alcohol during combat. When a rest period arrived, however, his recipe consisted of placing sweetened lemon powder into an aluminum canteen, adding some heavily chlorinated water from whatever source, and dosing that mixture with alcohol derived from the medical supplies. He called the awful concoction White Flash.

OKINAWA

Our Division's rest was limited, and we soon began loading ships for another battle. This time, although most of us did not know it until en route, we were headed for Okinawa. The Japanese were anticipating an attack on the southern tip of that long island, but MacArthur somehow assembled a huge fleet of ships that carried two Army infantry and two Marine divisions for a surprise attack about midway on Okinawa's west side. Evidently the Japanese were not well prepared for such an assault, and their main defense against our invasion consisted of dispatching kamikaze pilots on suicide missions to disrupt our landing. Scores of them attacked our ships, which the Japanese had apparently discovered approaching Okinawa only the night before our attack. Flying very cheap aircraft with only enough gasoline for a one-way journey, the kamikaze pilots were surrounded by huge amounts of explosives and expected to die while ramming their planes against our ships. Although violating the rule against observing such action, I managed, along with a few others, to watch the tremendous display of armament for a few minutes. Our anti-aircraft fire destroyed most of the planes flying toward us, although some did manage to hit a few ships.

Early on the morning of April 1, 1945, the four Marine and Army divisions landed abreast on Okinawa. Encountering little opposition on land, we made a rapid advance and within a few days our attack force controlled the central portion of the island. The Japanese could not turn their big guns around rapidly from the southern tip of the island where they had expected our landing. Later, of course, we encountered fierce opposition on Okinawa in one of the Pacific's bloodiest battles.

On the third day after the landing, however, we still had met no substantial enemy resistance, and so I resumed my role as preventive medicine officer. Pursuing my first priority (i.e., ascertaining the nature of local mosquitoes that might carry disease), I discovered some marsh water where they were breeding in a beautiful valley near our troop concentration. While bending over the water's edge to pick up and examine mosquito larvae in my dipper, I noticed two men coming down a hill into the valley and toward me. My initial thought, of course, was "Friend or foe?" Fortunately, I soon recognized that they were American soldiers.

Then I realized that my being in this situation violated several rules that could bring me into serious trouble. I was alone, which is absolutely prohibited in combat, and away from headquarters without permission. An officer must always keep his weapons close at hand, whereas my carbine and pistol were about fifty feet away. We did not wear metal insignia in combat because Japanese snipers selectively picked off officers, but close-up one could tell another's rank by the markings of insignia left on our fatigue uniforms. Thus I discerned that the two men were a corporal and a private, and they could see that I was a captain. Sensing that it would be highly desirable to defend my situation vigorously and that the best defense is a good offense, I gave them a mini-lecture on mosquito biology and the diseases that mosquitoes can carry. That included explaining that the larval stage precedes the adult flying insect, and that the larvae of anopheles mosquitoes, which carry malaria, lie at the water's surface in an almost horizontal position, whereas the larvae of mosquitoes carrying dengue fever lie in a slanting position with only one end contacting the water's surface. The men listened quietly. In fact, they did not say a word until, after about ten minutes, they turned and left. Before they were out of earshot, however, I heard one say to the other, " . . . and for Christ's sake they make guys officers for that." Thus I escaped penalty for violating so many Army rules.

The first few days on Okinawa turned out to be a quiet prelude to a very tough battle. Upon moving toward the south we encountered heavy Japanese forces of fierce fighters; our casualties became extensive and backlogged our surgical teams. Again, as on Leyte, I was pressed into shock tent service. One night a corporal and I were attending about fifteen seriously wounded soldiers who were lying on cots down the middle of the long shock tent awaiting surgical care. As the corporal bent over a soldier to place a needle into his vein, I observed a huge snake behind him, still dragging its tail from outside the tent and seemingly ready to strike his calf. Responding to my yell the corporal wheeled around; the reptile then passed directly under the cot on which the wounded soldier was lying and turned between the two lines of patients. We feared that the snake, whose five foot length we could now fully see, would strike a soldier. My associate grabbed a shovel and meeting the snake as it emerged from the lines of bloody wounded, he banged its head. We were immensely relieved after that brief but intense ordeal.

As generally seems to happen in the Army when an unusual incident occurs, experts suddenly appear. Among the small group of soldiers that quickly gathered around the battered snake, one identified the specimen as a hemi-habu, a highly poisonous species that was common in Okinawa. Opening the jaws and demonstrating with his finger, he pointed out that on one side the snake had an anomalous double-pronged fang (poison injector) but only the usual single prong on the other side. During the discussion after the "lecture," to our astonishment the snake began moving again. Someone quickly grabbed the shovel and chopped off its head. That reminded me of my own manual-prescribed duty: preserve in alcohol the head of any large snake found and send it to higher headquarters for study. Word of that experience spread rapidly, and during the ensuing days front-line soldiers found several such reptiles on the rocky ground over which they were advancing. The more enterprising men would cut off the snakes' heads, approach their commanding officers, and explain that "the doctor" back at division headquarters desperately needed them for submission to higher headquarters. Thus, they would escape the combat line for a few hours while delivering the booty. With many snakes' heads arriving in this fashion our dwindling supply of alcohol (only potable alcohol being available) aroused loud outcries from my fellow officers. We did not actually encounter any snake bites, and we did manage to preserve some alcohol for White Flash rather than pickling snakes' heads.

Meanwhile our Seventh Division as a whole was struggling mightily for the island, which the Japanese fervently defended. After turning their big guns around, they pounded us as we moved from Okinawa's midpoint toward the south. The battle became a major turning point in the tide against Japan, clearly a prelude to attacking the core of Japan itself.

By that time Hitlerism had been defeated in Europe and May 12, 1945, had been designated as Victory in Europe (VE) Day, so our nation's war effort could now be concentrated on bringing down the Japanese military machine. Though battered and retreating, the latter remained formidable. Despite our realization that some of us would be the last American casualties in the war, it was exhilarating to know that we were winning; the Seventh Division leadership had instilled fierce pride in us.

Using Casualties of One Epidemic to Fight Another

As the Division proceeded to fight its way south we encountered not only further heavy casualties but two additional epidemics. One was dengue fever, a severe and disabling mosquito-borne disease characterized by fever, severe backache, headache, and fatigue. Usually recovery occurs in about ten to fifteen days, but during that time the pain becomes so tormenting that the patient sometimes expresses concern not that he is going to die but that he is *not* going to die. Because that epidemic was disabling many of our soldiers, I approached the Division commander, General "Vinegar Joe" Stilwell, to seek a detail of men who would accompany me into semi-forward areas, just behind advancing troops, to spray the larval breeding sites with DDT—mostly pots of water around the newly abandoned, walled clusters of huts where the Okinawans had lived prior to the battle. I explained to the General how we must stop the mosquitoes that transmit the dengue fever virus by spraying the larvae and thus minimize casualties from the epidemic. Violating instructions, I had managed to get some DDT and knapsack sprayers loaded for the Okinawa invasion. To my plan, however, the General responded in language indicating how he had acquired the nickname, "Vinegar Joe." He made it utterly clear that my request was the most ludicrous proposal he had ever heard and that in our situation every man was needed behind a real weapon to kill Japanese soldiers, not a DDT spray gun to kill mosquitoes.

A few days before the dengue fever outbreak, a second epidemic—battle fatigue—had also struck the Division, with lassitude as its major symptom. Although it had been taking a huge toll in Europe, battle fatigue had not previously affected Pacific Theater troops extensively. But when we encountered heavy artillery from the guns turned on us as we moved south, scores of our men suffered battle fatigue. The treatment consisted of relieving them from combat temporarily, holding them at the clearing station, and then moving them forward again as soon as sufficient recovery permitted and before they became too accustomed to freedom from front-line conditions.

The situation gave me an idea. I spoke to the psychiatrist in charge of the battle fatigue patients: "I understand you want the men to go forward as they improve but not immediately into combat." "That's right," he replied. I proposed that he assign a few such men to me so that I could train them for DDT spraying and then have them accompany me into the villages up ahead as we took them. He agreed that the plan would combine psychiatric treatment with preventive medicine and thus find a way around a higher echelon decision that obstructed a task that circumstances required (The venture ultimately induced the General to recommend me for a Bronze Star!). Some days later, as my crew and I entered one of the villages, we encountered unexpected machine gun fire from inside the deserted compound. Our men quickly captured a lone enemy soldier somehow left behind by the retreating Japanese forces. Questioned about why he opened fire rather than laying low until we passed, he explained that he had thought we were coming after him with flame-throwers rather than our knapsack DDT sprayers.

THE ATOM BOMB

I remember clearly the evening of August 6, 1945—Hiroshima Day. We had secured Okinawa through heavy combat, and after working all day loading for the obvious assault on the main body of Japan we were becoming highly conscious of the huge numbers of casualties expected there. Heavy resistance with tremendous firepower would confront us, essentially like what happened in the Normandy invasion. Gathered around a small radio for the evening newscast a small group of us learned about the first atom-bomb blast and its huge civilian toll. The obvious implications provoked my life's most mixed sensation, and I suspect that of my companions. We realized with relief that the likelihood of our being killed while invading Japan had been virtually eliminated, but killing so many Hiroshima civilians as the price made us distraught. It was a torturing, wonderful-terrible feeling. More than a half-century later I still reflect on the personal feelings of having avoided an invasion of central Japan mixed with appreciating the military rationale that maximum terror should be inflicted on the enemy, but greatly shocked at destroying a whole city of essentially noncombatant people. About the only thing that gives me some comfort is the satisfaction of having been a soldier in helping bring down the Hitler-Hirohito axis.

KOREA

We continued loading ships, but the Division's destination was changed to Inchon, the port city for Seoul, Korea. With peace just established, I did not then realize the political significance of our landing in what eventually became South Korea. Relieved of invading Japan, we were just happy to be somewhere else and out of combat.

The first afternoon at Inchon I happened to disembark with a Special Services officer who invited me to join him in his jeep. Touring the strangely peaceful countryside we observed an inn nestled in some low hills. As we approached and entered, a retinue of attendants escorted us to a single table set lavishly for about six persons but apparently meant just for our arrival! Briefly wandering about the establishment while awaiting our meal my companion noticed a bottle of Scotch whisky, something we had not seen in a long while. Quickly responding to our interest, an attendant opened the bottle and poured us substantial drinks. We were thoroughly jolted a half hour later, however, just as we were thoroughly enjoying the situation, and dinner seemed about ready. Two other jeeps carrying several high army and navy brass rolled up to the inn's entrance; the local people had obviously mistaken the major and me as early arrivals for a really important party. After surrendering what was left of the whisky we were allowed to eat a much lesser meal in a different room from that of the real party.

A few days after our arrival in Korea in August 1945, we all began calculating the time when we could return home. The army had devised a scheme that set the date for return according to the number of points that had been earned by months of military service in the war, including extra points for months overseas and for the number of children born no later than VE Day. My second son, Jack, had been born in 1944 while our family was in San Francisco, and my third, Stephen, entered the world precisely on VE Day, thus providing the points necessary to get me home a few months early.

The return by ship necessitated a transfer in Manila, where I decided to have a grand meal before leaving the Orient. During the third course in a great hotel with a magnificent, old dining room, a huge rat traveling along a dripping pipe immediately overhead destroyed the ambience and my taste for the meal. It was also a symbol of the huge tasks that confronted public health now that the war was over. The next day I boarded ship for the voyage back to San Francisco.

THE IDEOLOGY OF WAR

Now, almost sixty years after my World War II experience and having observed how war has changed since that time, I realize that the twentieth century transformed the nature of international combat, not only in weaponry but also in its globalization. From its beginnings in primitive tribal conflict over land (economy) and hegemony, war has extended to reflect nationalism and has moved into international alliances. Yet its social roots seem much the same.

The human instinct for control over resources has unfolded through various configurations into modern capitalism as the dominant form of society in the early twenty-first century. A highly significant aspect of that development has been the concentration of wealth into the hands of a relatively few people in the most powerful countries, and that power has passed into the hands of those countries' political leaders who act on the international scene. Meanwhile, vast numbers of people have been left in poverty. Those in the most impoverished nations become enraged at their lack of control over the world's obvious resources as well as those in their own countries. Their rage is increasingly and sometimes violently directed at the dominating nations of the world. Meanwhile, the powerful have become practically oblivious to the situation they are creating while enlarging their domination over the world's resources. In the endeavor to control land, oil, minerals, and other commodities as well as trade, people matter only as a means of such control.

This fundamental phenomenon is intimately linked to ideology. Tribalism-nationalism generates patriotic allegiance that rises sharply whenever the group is threatened, and that notion is enhanced by the idea of "my group's innate superiority." That idea is quite readily manipulated even among so-called well-educated people, as exemplified by Hitler's generating the Nazi view of Aryan supremacy among Germans in the 1930s that led to the Holocaust. The concept of supremacy still prevails widely in the world. It could be observed when U.S. soldiers referred to the Okinawans as "gooks" whose lives were not worth much; they were just "in the way" of defeating Japan. That might not have been official policy, but the notion was widely expressed in soldier talk.

Religious fervor is another important element in war ideology: "My god is all-powerful and must be recognized as such; the infidels must be overcome." From the Christian crusades to the Moslem Al-Qaeda and right-wing Israeli nationalism, that belief has motivated people to war. Suicide attacks can become the standard of loyalty in battle; kamikaze pilots showed their devotion to Emperor Hirohito that way, and it is the way Al-Qaeda adherents show their devotion to Allah.

The escalating power of modern weaponry has vastly increased warfare's potential for damage. Land mines, atomic bombs, biological and chemical means of attack, missiles, and satellite communication strengthen the capacity for waging war and even committing genocide. National leaders currently possess immense power to use weaponry, as in the case of Truman's decision to use the atomic bomb against Hiroshima and Nagasaki. Were both necessary, or even one? We will never know, although we may have strong feelings about the matter. Did Johnson's decision to continue bombing North Vietnam really support America's genuine interest? In historical perspective the answer to that question increasingly seems "no." Will the Nazi extermination ovens or the recent airplane strikes against prominent American buildings be repeated, or even more horrible forms of human destruction be invented?

Avoiding these latter prospects obviously rests upon humanity's capacity to formulate and implement ways of minimizing conflict among peoples and ultimately rooting out its sources. That entails overcoming the massive gaps in wealth within and between nations and dealing seriously with the ideological forces that are intertwined with and augment the economic forces of our times, for example, in Iraq. Although the United Nations, Amnesty International, and like-minded organizations are tackling some important current issues, it is by no means clear that we are nearing a universal commitment to achieve peace in the world. Perhaps international courts are a primitive beginning to overcome the deficiencies in mankind's development that lead to war. As long as we tolerate and even encourage further accumulation of wealth by billionaires and their corporations in Saudi Arabia, the United States, and elsewhere in the face of massive world-wide poverty, I do not understand how we can hope to achieve peace. Private profit may currently be essential for efficient productivity, but it must be democratically and effectively controlled to minimize its adverse consequences.

What some of us regard as terrorists others see as rebels; it is a matter of perspective. I hope, in the interest of peace, we can deal with the realities that generate such perspectives.

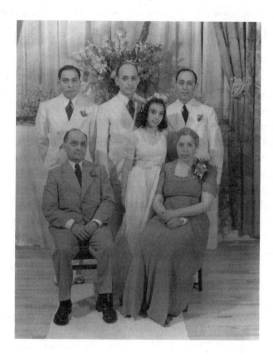

Breslow family, circa 1939. Front (l to r): father Joseph Breslow, mother Mayme Breslow. Middle: sister Shirley Breslow. Rear (l to r): Brothers Sidney Breslow, Lester Breslow, Arthur Breslow.

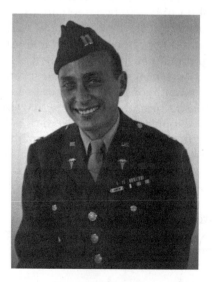

Captain Lester Breslow, 1945.

Disease Control

4

Modern public health originated as a social movement to combat the urban epidemics that were threatening nineteenth-century industrialization and economic development. As factories opened, rural people flocked into the cities, where they worked long hours under harsh conditions and lived in crowded homes with inadequate food in unsanitary communities. At the start of the twentieth century these conditions still resulted in repeated epidemics of the common respiratory and gastrointestinal diseases and particularly heavy loads of tuberculosis and pneumonia/influenza. Each of the latter caused about one-tenth of all deaths in the United States, making them lead the mortality list. Tuberculosis, then known as "The Captain of the Men of Death," brought about 30 percent of all deaths among persons 15–60 years of age. The third leading cause of death in 1900 was diarrhea and enteritis, which at that time was diagnosed mainly as dysentery.

While living in Bismarck during the early 1920s, my brothers and I suffered measles and chicken pox, which people and their physicians then accepted as inevitable diseases of childhood. The particularly prolonged cough that followed my encounter with whooping cough induced my mother to push me into what I now recognize as alternative medicine. She learned the remedy from neighbors, namely, breathing from a pot of hot tar an hour or two a day for several days. Although intended to alleviate the cough, in retrospect I realize that this treatment may have been my heaviest exposure to respiratory carcinogens. Medical science had not yet produced the means for artificial immunity against the common respiratory infections of childhood.

Besides these relatively minor conditions that affected nearly every child during the early part of the century, more severe diseases also spread widely. Smallpox epidemics still occurred, as did outbreaks of scarlet fever, at the time a common streptococcal infection accompanied by a rash. Rheumatic fever in childhood, which was later recognized as another streptococcal infection, frequently left its victims with damaged heart valves, which often led to heart enlargement and early death. That disease, though common, was not even recognized as a public health problem in the classic textbook of public health that appeared in 1914 (Rosenau, 1914). Diarrheal disease, including the well-defined typhoid fever but commonly caused by other organisms as well, took a tremendous toll. Usually a consequence of contaminated water or food, it attacked youngsters and elderly people most severely because of their vulnerability to the dehydration that accompanied diarrhea.

Poliomyelitis, in those days generally called infantile paralysis and recognized as communicable, appeared in texts under a miscellaneous rubric because the specific organism causing it and the mode of transmission were not clear. Though first diagnosed in the eighteenth century, the disease evidently began increasing considerably during the early part of the twentieth. Until a vaccine was developed, parents greatly feared that their children might encounter poliomyelitis during the late summer months when it usually occurred.

The group of conditions designated as venereal diseases in the early part of the century and now known as sexually transmitted diseases (STD) could not be mentioned in "polite" society. Surgeon General Thomas Parran first used the word *syphilis* on the radio in 1936 to finally break the taboo. In the United States, malaria, whose mosquito transmission Ross had discovered in 1895, was the most prevalent insect-borne disease and it imposed an especially heavy burden in the southeastern states (Rosenau, 1914). People also commonly combated flies and other disease-carrying insects in an effort to keep such diseases at bay.

When I entered public health in the mid-twentieth century, the communicable diseases still dominated the public health agenda. Tuberculosis had declined considerably, largely due to improvements in the general standard of living (McKeown, 1976). Our public health aim in tuberculosis control then was to increase the ratio of cases to deaths by finding the patients as early as possible in the course of their disease, and then trying with rest and good nutrition to achieve recoveries. Smallpox still sometimes affected American communities (as well as others throughout the world) even though vaccination had been shown to be effective a century and a half previously. Against diphtheria, a then common respiratory and sometimes fatal disease among children, we used both toxoid to prevent infection and antitoxin for youngsters already infected but not yet significantly harmed by the bacilli; improvement by mid-century, however, still left thousands of cases occurring each year in the United States.

When drugs for effective therapy became available (first the sulfonamides for treatment of certain bacterial infections and then penicillin) the new pharmaceuticals proved so powerful against a wide array of diseases caused by bacteria that they received popular acclaim as the "wonder drugs." Chemotherapy markedly reduced mortality from pneumonia and other communicable diseases as well as morbidity from gonorrhea and other conditions that had resisted previously available treatment.

The second half of the twentieth century also ushered in a new era of vaccines against viral and bacterial infections. I recall two personal episodes involving vaccines. Shortly after the Salk vaccine had been proven effective against the much-dreaded poliomyelitis in 1955, and the inactivated polio virus vaccine came onto the market, I noticed that the drug store window near our State Department of Public Health office in Berkeley, where I was then employed, displayed an advertisement for it. Believing that the vaccine distribution was still restricted to a few special groups, I mentioned my observation to colleagues working in acute communicable disease control. When they assured me that a small amount was being allowed into regular commercial channels, I rushed back and purchased enough for my three sons, who were then 10–15 years old, the age when polio commonly occurred. At home I placed the brown bag containing the vials of vaccine in the refrigerator, but after a few days my wife insisted that I remove the bag because she worried that "it might contaminate the food." So I announced to my sons that everyone must be home at four P.M. the next day, April 26, 1955, to visit our doctor for the shots. Despite their wailing about missing sports and other planned after-school activities I demanded their attendance. The next day, however, I learned about the "Cutter incident," the several poliomyelitis cases that occurred among persons vaccinated with that company's product. The vaccine, my colleagues told me, evidently contained some live virus particles that were supposed to have been killed, and several persons inoculated with that company's vaccine had developed poliomyelitis two weeks thereafter, the usual incubation time. Public announcement that the Cutter vaccine should not be used and was being withdrawn from the market was not yet being made, so I could not bring the restricted information home. Therefore, I simply delayed my arrival home (amid heavy family complaint). Upon inspection of the brown bag's contents I discovered that the vaccine came from the same lot as that involved in the Cutter cases. The incident taught me the lesson, "Be not the first by whom the new is tried, now yet the last to lay the old aside."

My second personal vaccine experience occurred in 1966 when I was California State Health Director. That year we suffered a rather severe outbreak of influenza. When newspaper reporters approached Governor "Pat" Brown about it, he responded, "Where's my Health Director?" I was found in a motel en route from Sacramento to Berkeley, too sick with influenza to complete the auto trip home. Several days later at a news conference one reporter asked, "Dr. Breslow, did you take the flu vaccine"? (The vaccine was then recommended for health personnel as well as for older people.) After a relatively long pause, because the answer, unfortunately, was "no," a young staff epidemiologist blurted out, "Dr. Breslow was in the control group." That brought down the house and thus averted damage to my reputation. Lesson: always keep bright staff people around.

The communicable disease challenge had actually decreased substantially from its peak during the early part of the century. Tuberculosis, though still accounting for more than 40,000 deaths each year in the United States, was steadily being overcome by improved living conditions, aided by the prevailing public health measures. Diarrheal diseases were yielding to better community and household sanitation. Specific immunizing agents were emerging as effective means of preventing not only diphtheria but also other communicable diseases. Data for California shown in Table 1 illustrate this trend.

During the second half of the twentieth century the world-wide eradication of smallpox and the reduction of poliomyelitis to the zero point in North and South America and some other parts of the world highlighted the further substantial progress against communicable conditions. The improvements, however, do not mean that communicable disease control is anywhere near complete. Such conditions still plague countries in the developing world; malaria and tuberculosis, for example, remain huge problems in many countries. Moreover, in the United States and other "advanced" nations as well as in the rest of the world, new communicable diseases are appearing, for example, HIV-AIDS and SARS, that public health must deal with.

MATERNAL AND CHILD HEALTH

Maternal and child health (MCH) is another highly significant area of public health progress. Concern about child health arose from the appalling conditions of child labor in some early factories and their consequences, against which social activists first expressed concern. Public health officially entered that field with passage of the national Shep-

TABLE 1   Percentage of All Deaths from Selected Communicable Diseases—California 1910–1950 (By place of occurrence 1910–1940, by place of residence 1950)

Cause of Death	Percentage of All Deaths				
	1910	1920	1930	1940	1950
Total, selected communicable disease causes of death	30.3	30.1	18.6	10.8	4.9
Selected communicable disease causes of death					
Tuberculosis	15.2	11.8	8.5	4.8	2.3
Pneumonia and influenza	7.6	12.1	7.2	5.1	2.0
Diarrhea and enteritis[a]	3.8	3.3	1.6	0.6	0.5
Specific acute communicable diseases[b]	3.7	2.9	1.3	0.3	0.1

[a]Gastritis, duodenitis, enteritis, and colitis, 1950
[b]Typhoid fever, scarlet fever, whooping cough, diphtheria, measles
Source: United States Public Health Service, National Office of Vital Statistics. California Department of Public Health (1965). Death Records Report CASDPH 1961–63

pard-Towner Act of 1921, which provided funds for state and local health department services to pregnant women and their offspring. Though opposed by much of the medical profession as an intrusion into its clinical medicine prerogatives and accused of wrongly expanding public health medical services beyond dealing with communicable diseases, MCH rapidly took root in governmental public health work. With federal support and guidance from the U.S. Children's Bureau, state and local agencies developed prenatal services, particularly for pregnant women who did not have access to private physicians, and undertook widespread education of women as well as physicians regarding standards of care for pregnant women. Child health clinics also became available to women and children with low incomes.

Although a clinical focus on infections, hemorrhage, and toxemias of pregnancy had to be maintained, reducing maternal mortality through routine medical and nursing care during pregnancy became the dominant theme of prenatal care. Regularly observing the blood pressure and weight, measuring the pelvis, and other services aimed at maintaining health inaugurated a new way of approaching health generally. It was a sharp break from the previous limitation among medical practitioners of providing "complaint–response" medicine and disease-specific preventive services. The new child health routines aimed not only at detecting and treating impairments, but also at adequate nutrition, establishing immunity, and good hygiene.

Thus MCH services launched public health participation into a new medical field, namely, to sustain health while people were "normal" and not merely to diagnose, treat, and sometimes seek to prevent disease. Although some medical leaders had long proposed that idea, their advocacy had not achieved its incorporation into regular practice. Unfortunately, beyond MCH services, health maintenance did not immediately become a substantial element of medical practice; only in recent years have health maintenance services become routine for more people.

Meanwhile, maternal mortality has declined 99 percent from its frequency at the beginning of the century, to the point where it is no longer included in routine health statistics. Infant mortality, too, has fallen dramatically in the United States, from 161 per 1000 live births in 1900 to 29 in 1950 and only seven at the end of the century. Not only have medical services aided that advance, but improved education, better standards of living, and several specific environmental measures based on scientific advances (such as pasteurized milk and safer water supplies) have contributed probably as much or more. However, maternal and infant mortality statistics in the United States still bring the country far down on the list of industrialized nations with respect to those key health indices. This is due in considerable part to the relatively slow improvement in maternal and infant mortality rates among African-American women, and is one of the reasons the United States Surgeon General has recently declared reduction of health disparities to be a major goal of national health policy.

THE BASIS FOR CHRONIC DISEASE CONTROL

Whereas the three leading causes of death in 1900 were tuberculosis, pneumonia-influenza, and diarrhea-enteritis, by 1945 heart disease, cancer, and cerebrovascular disease topped the list. These latter three conditions, which had been responsible for less than one-fifth of all deaths in the United States at the beginning of the century, accounted for more than half at mid-century. From 1900 to the mid-1940s heart disease had become the leading disease causing death and the cancer mortality rate had risen by 50 percent; lung cancer alone was soon to overtake tuberculosis as a cause of death.

Selected data for the United States concerning chronic disease mortality during the period 1910–1950, which appear in Table 2, emphasize the major trends during that period. Whereas tuberculosis deaths declined to

TABLE 2   Death Rates for Selected Causes of Death, United States, 1900 and 1950

Cause of Death	1900 Rate per 100,000	Cause of Death	1950 Rate per 100,000
All causes	1719	All causes	964
Pneumonia, influenza	202	Heart disease	356
Tuberculosis	194	Cancer	140
Diarrhea, enteritis	143	Vascular lesions of CNS	104
Heart disease	137	Pneumonia, influenza	31
Intracranial lesions	107	Tuberculosis	23
Cancer	64		

Source: National Office of Vital Statistics, *Vital Statistics of the U.S. 1950*, Vol. I, p. 209.

one-eighth of their earlier level, and other communicable disease mortality also fell sharply, cancer deaths doubled and those from heart disease almost tripled. Heart disease deaths by 1950 accounted for more than one-third of all deaths and cancer for one-seventh.

Clearly, the chronic diseases had become the major health problem. It was commonly believed, however, that they were an inevitable consequence of an aging population. Physicians and others regarded them as degenerative diseases; people living into their sixties and seventies simply had to expect some, often fatal, chronic disease. Lack of a morbidity system precluded understanding that more than three-fourths of the chronic disease cases actually started among persons 15–64 years old. Meanwhile, public health still remained largely geared to communicable disease control activities.

On board ship en route back from the Pacific after World War II, and still strongly committed to a public health career, I had spent considerable time considering what should be done for health (including chronic disease control) during the next several decades and how my career could be relevant. Action regarding the chronic diseases seemed to rest largely in the welfare domain because the health sector at that time could do so little about them. Pessimism about the situation prevailed. The chronic diseases struck poor people more frequently than they did the affluent, and income loss due to disability and treatment costs often led to impoverishment. Social policies shunted many chronically ill persons into almshouses, county farms, and other institutions that had fancier names but were not much different in nature. In effect, pushing the victims "out of sight, out of mind" constituted the social policy. The prospect of using scientific advances to overcome or prevent chronic disease and its consequences was largely neglected.

But some progress actually had been made. Twenty-five years previously a diagnosis of diabetes or pernicious anemia had usually meant a lingering death sentence. By the 1940s, however, persons with those diseases whose conditions were detected early and properly treated could anticipate an almost normal longevity. The likelihood of coping effectively with the increasing cancer and cardiovascular disease burdens nevertheless still seemed remote.

Stirrings against these negative attitudes did emerge. Progressive physician and hospital leaders began to insist that a community's general medical resources should provide more aggressive services for the chronically ill (Boas, 1947). They advocated incorporating such patients into the medical mainstream rather than sending them to separate facilities where they would be largely neglected. Also, some physicians became increasingly enthusiastic about what they could accomplish for specific disease problems such as cancer. Beginning in the early half of the century they recruited prominent laymen for an attack on that disease. These activities were becoming highly successful, attracting large private contributions for research and patient services, and lobbying for congressional appropriations for research. For example, as early as 1913 a group of gynecological surgeons had formed the American Society for the Control of Cancer, later to become the American Cancer Society.

State and federal governments likewise began to take action. The Massachusetts legislature, in 1926, authorized the state health department to plan for cancer patient care. In 1937 Congress passed an act establishing the National Cancer Institute (NCI) and the National Advisory Cancer Council, for the purpose of

> conducting researches [*sic*], investigations, experiments and studies relating to the causes, diagnosis and treatment of cancer; assisting and fostering similar research activities by other agencies, public and private; and promoting the coordination of all such researches and activities and the useful application of their results with a view to the development and prompt widespread use of the most effective methods of prevention, diagnosis and treatment of cancer. [The National Cancer Institute Act (1937)].

Although the National Cancer Institute has brilliantly carried out the first two mandates, it has failed in the third. Basic and clinical scientists essentially captured the institution and managed to devote its resources almost exclusively to their exciting opportunities. Thus, despite great achievements in research the NCI made little effort apart from training some physicians toward "the useful application of their results," as specified in the legislation. It has left that matter, particularly prevention, to others, and that policy has resulted in a tremendous lag in cancer control. For example, methods of detecting, diagnosing, and treating cervical cancer effectively were well established by 1950. Yet for the next quarter century approximately 10,000 women in the United States continued to die annually from that one type of cancer, a total of about 250,000 during 1950–1975. And during the century's last quarter approximately 5,000 deaths occurred each year, for another 125,000. Yet, because the deaths occurred one by one rather than in clusters known as epidemics, the problem was largely neglected. Imagine the outcry if smallpox had continued to cause such devastation.

During the mid-century period attacks on other chronic diseases through programs sponsored by dedicated physicians, voluntary health organizations, and government gained support. Thus, the American Heart Association appeared, along with the National Heart Institute (which was later to become the National Heart, Lung, and Blood Institute). Several other comparable pairs of voluntary health organizations and National Institutes of Health appeared and have become important elements in the American approach to research on the chronic diseases, but the emphasis on basic and clinical science and the relative neglect of aggressiveness in applying knowledge of control measures has continued. To some extent the Centers for Disease Control and Prevention (CDC) has picked up the challenge; however, its budget for doing so is tiny compared to that of the NIH. That imbalance has not been addressed, especially if it is assumed that the responsibility for chronic disease control lies with the CDC.

The idea that chronic disease might be largely prevented attracted little early attention. Knowledge of how to do that remained meager and awaited the substantial epidemiological research that was just starting at mid-century. The concept that an increasing chronic disease burden inevitably accompanied an aging population and that there was no role for public health continued to prevail. Nevertheless, some of us pointed out that opportunities abounded for incorporating chronic disease control interests into several well-established public health activities. For example, traditional public health statistical services could be expanded beyond concern with births, deaths, and communicable diseases to include attention to the incidence of, and mortality from, chronic diseases. Epidemiologists could investigate the circumstances that lead to their occurrence. Public health nursing could enlarge its scope to include such patients as well as those with communicable and pre- and post-natal problems. Health education could likewise extend its focus to cover emerging knowledge of what can be done about the chronic diseases.

I believed strongly that fulfilling the public health mission in the post-World War II period required tackling the chronic disease problem vigorously and comprehensively. Three ideas occurred to me. One was that we should begin maintaining surveillance over the nature and extent of the several chronic diseases, and particularly the trends in their incidence, prevalence, and fatality among different segments of the population. Such measurement data would provide a basis for epidemiological study of the problem and ultimately guide control programs. Essentially, the only information about the problem at the time came from death certificates. While helpful, such data did not suffice because the public health interest required including consideration of the vast amount of chronic disease morbidity and disability as well as the deaths. With the prevailing medical circumstances and information technology it obviously would be impractical to expect physicians to report chronic diseases in the same manner that they reported communicable diseases. How then could the necessary data be assembled? That question had to be answered.

My second thought was simply to incorporate into governmental public health activity, and thus extend, what voluntary health agencies such as the American Cancer Society were already doing about the problem. They were promoting early disease detection to make treatment more effective by encouraging knowledge of cancer symptoms and prompt action by people and their physicians whenever such symptoms appeared. Efforts aimed at early detection could be enhanced using new screening technology, for example, the already available Papanicolaou smear for cervical cancer. It seemed likely that comparable means would be developed and should be applied for discovering other forms of cancer in their early stages as well as heart disease, diabetes, and other chronic conditions, especially among segments of the population where epidemiologic evidence indicated that such action was most needed. It would be necessary, of course, to educate physicians and the general public to support such endeavors and promote check-ups to detect disease among people who were still apparently well, before symptoms appeared but after asymptomatic pathologic changes had started.

Third, whereas preventing chronic diseases by discovering and combating microbic causes seemed very unlikely, possibilities concerning other preventive measures such as avoiding obesity and certain occupational exposures were already evident. Louis Dublin, a Metropolitan Life Insurance Company actuary, had demonstrated in the 1930s that obesity strongly predicted and therefore seemed to have a causative relationship to early mortality (Dublin, 1949). Toxicologists and epidemiologists had identified benzene and other chemicals to which industrial workers were exposed as factors in cancer. Such knowledge was growing and seemed likely to expand rapidly through developing and applying epidemiological methods that had proved useful in delineating the causes of pellagra and some other chronic conditions.

The time appeared ripe to overcome the prevailing notion that the chronic diseases were degenerative, that is, inevitable consequences of aging. Even a preventive approach to them seemed feasible, though beyond the traditional lines of approach that experience with communicable diseases had fostered. Such ideas did not, of course, originate in a vacuum. They grew in part out of simply applying to the chronic diseases what had already been learned in public health: (1) using epidemiology as the basic tool for delineating disease problems; (2) identifying cases and providing treatment for patients before extensive damage occurred, paralleling approaches to tuberculosis and syphilis; and (3) finding and applying means of prevention. The nascent campaign against cancer encouraged such a triadic effort.

ENTRY TO THE CALIFORNIA DEPARTMENT OF PUBLIC HEALTH

Arriving in San Francisco back from military service as 1945 was ending, I was determined to remain in California rather than return to Minnesota. The family situation favored it; my wife had been born there and her parents still lived in California. The State Department of Public Health, which enjoyed an excellent reputation under Wilton Halverson as the State Director of Public Health and Governor Earl Warren, seemed a good place to start a chronic disease program. California was already undergoing its postwar readjustment, which entailed building schools, hospitals, and other institutions that had been relatively neglected during the early 1940s. Due to immigration, the population of approximately nine million California residents in 1946 was increasing rapidly, and they required expanding public services to meet their needs.

Appreciating the possible influence of using the contact that I had made with Dr. Karl Meyer during my military stint at the San Francisco Port of Embarkation, I asked him to introduce me to Dr. Halverson. Dr. Meyer responded by telephoning Dr. Halverson immediately, but was apparently told that Dr. Halverson would call him back. Dr. Meyer exploded into the phone and insisted upon talking to Dr. Halverson "right now." Then, putting his hand over the mouthpiece, he explained to me, "When I want to talk with Dr. Halverson, I talk with Dr. Halverson." It was evident that Dr. Halverson would have to see me.

I went to see him the next day, well prepared, I thought, with a twenty-minute speech on why public health should tackle the chronic diseases.

Halverson sat at the corner of his desk with his chin cupped in his hand, listening intently. After about five minutes into the statement I realized from his stony face that he was completely rejecting my proposal and I thought that perhaps some dialogue might improve the prospects. I paused. Halverson simply glared at me for a long time and finally said, "Dr. Breslow, why don't you go back to Minnesota and try out those ideas there?" He was obviously reflecting the prevailing view among public health leaders that health departments should stick to their traditional activities: communicable disease control, including associated laboratory service; environmental health; maternal and child health; health education; and vital statistics. Health departments should avoid any move toward the noncommunicable diseases because taking such steps might provoke conflict with organized medicine. The latter carried considerable political clout and had accepted, even advocated, public health efforts to prevent and control communicable disease epidemics, but strongly resisted any public health efforts that might, they worried, "take patients away" from them. What could be done about the chronic diseases anyway except to treat the patients the way physicians were doing?

After that disappointing encounter with Halverson a family vacation seemed like a good idea. Returning from that vacation, back in San Francisco and beginning to pack for the return to Minnesota, I went to say good-bye to a colleague, Dr. Jessica Bierman, who was then Chief of the Maternal and Child Health Bureau in the California Department of Public Health. We had met through a mutual friend. Upon learning of my situation Dr. Bierman insisted that I see Dr. Robert Dyar, who had just been recruited to head the Department's Division of Preventive Medical Services, which embraced the several medical bureaus concerned with prevention, such as Dr. Bierman's. Accordingly, I did see Dr. Dyar and advanced the same notions that I had prepared for Halverson. Dyar listened to the whole of the presentation and at its conclusion, after a few polite words of commendation, he asked, "Do you know anything about encephalitis?" To that disconcerting question I replied that nobody knew much about that disease, but that I had had some experience in two small encephalitis outbreaks, one in Minnesota and the other in Okinawa. Dyar expressed great enthusiasm and offered me the opportunity to lead an encephalitis study that the California State Legislature had just mandated. Concerned about the spread of equine encephalitis among humans as well as horses in California's San Joaquin Valley, the Legislature had just appropriated $200,000 (a huge sum for a public health study in those days) to conduct the project. Dyar emphasized the project's great importance and the Legislature's support. I thanked him for his consideration, but stated flatly that I wanted to pursue chronic disease as a public health endeavor and had little interest in encephalitis. He then offered a compromise: that I undertake the study of encephalitis, but on field visits to the small towns hit by the epidemic, where there were no very good restaurants and no entertainment, I should spend evenings in the motels writing my ideas about how public health could approach chronic disease control. When I asked if he would read such communications Dr. Dyar insisted that he would read them and, in fact, give the ideas serious consideration.

That compromise—an immediate position and the invitation to propose a public health approach to the chronic diseases—was acceptable to me because I was convinced that an opportunity would develop somehow to tackle them as a public health problem. The encephalitis work entailed seeing physicians and their patients in the San Joaquin Valley where I followed Dyar's advice, writing every evening what I thought public health should be doing about the chronic diseases, in addition to reports concerning the encephalitis cases that I had seen during the day. Although our departmental study yielded very little, during that same period William Hammond and William Reeves at the University of California in San Francisco were demonstrating that mosquitoes carried the disease and thus opened the path to control.

Whenever I was in the Department's San Francisco headquarters during early 1946 while pursuing the encephalitis problem, the possibility of encountering Halverson in the hallways and being thrown out of the Department worried me so greatly that I would actually watch the corridors carefully when going to the restroom in order to avoid meeting the stern Director and his wrath when he discovered that the man he sent away had returned through the back door. In June 1946, the dreaded call from Halverson summoned me to his office. Fortunately, however, that encounter did not confirm my fear. Instead, Halverson asked me to accompany him the next day to take charge of the poliomyelitis epidemic that was then severely hitting Los Angeles. The occurrence of many paralytic cases was understandably arousing great public alarm, but there was essentially nothing we could really do about it from the public health standpoint except keep track of the epidemic. Attending physicians were also helpless beyond providing comfort and arranging for an "iron lung" in case of respiratory failure. The situation brought to mind the old clinical-medical adage about dealing with critically ill patients for whom no known procedures would be useful: "Don't just do something, stand there!" So in epidemics where no known active measures can be helpful, the public health official must "just stand there."

In Los Angeles Halverson spent a few hours with me explaining specifically what being in charge of the epidemic meant. As he was leaving on vacation for a couple of weeks, the first thing I had to do was to drive around the city in his big, black automobile so that people would know the state health officer was monitoring the situation and doing what he could. That involved maneuvering his car out of the state building's basement garage, around the huge cement columns that supported the building but seriously impeded vehicular movement in the garage. Thus a critical element of the task was assuring that the big, black automobile would suffer no scratch from the pillars. Second, Halverson took me to meet Arthur Will, Director of the Los Angeles County Department of Charities, which then included the local public hospital system. On the way to Will's office Halverson emphasized that I must make everyone understand that the State Department of Public Health, and not Arthur Will, was in charge of the epidemic. Upon encountering Arthur Will's dominating personality I immediately understood the second directive but accepted the challenge only because Halverson strongly insisted that I must assume the leadership for public health being in charge of the epidemic. Third, Halverson instructed me to maintain contact with the county hospital physicians who were treating most of the patients to ensure that cases were being properly reported. That task acquainted me with John Affeldt, a rehabilitation expert who was doing the most constructive work during the epidemic, that is, organizing and directing care for about 100 patients at home in iron lungs. His arrangements entailed not only the necessary medical services but also maintaining standby generators in case the electricity-operated iron lungs should suffer power loss.

It was an exciting summer. Among other things I learned a bit about how public health deals with the press, particularly to be clear and emphatic. The information presented to the media consisted largely of the numbers and trends of cases that physicians throughout the county reported to the health department. I was thus able to assert "authority" and thwart Arthur Will's tendency to seize the limelight.

THE BUREAU OF CHRONIC DISEASE

In August, while still in charge of the Los Angeles poliomyelitis epidemic, I received a telephone call from Dyar informing me that Congress had allocated some funds specifically for cancer control that the National Cancer Institute was distributing to the states. That reflected Congressional intent that the NCI carry out the third function of the original (1937) Act, i.e., to apply research results to cancer control; though the Institute showed little enthusiasm, it did demonstrate some compliance by transmitting funds to the states. Dyar wanted me to start a cancer control program but readily assented to our establishing a departmental unit not just for that purpose as some states were doing but rather a Bureau of Chronic Disease. Perhaps those memos from the San Joaquin Valley during the early part of the year had helped persuade him that we would next be tackling heart disease, stroke, diabetes, and other chronic diseases, and that our approach to them would be similar to what we would be doing about cancer.

Beginning the new program was interrupted by still another brief communicable disease assignment, this one to assist the Berkeley City Health Officer vaccinate people in that community who were concerned about the possible spread of smallpox from Washington state where a few cases of the disease had occurred. Outside the Berkeley City Hall the local, well-seasoned health officer taught me how to vaccinate long lines of people on the sidewalk using his chisel method rather than the standard needle. A few light turns of a small chisel into the skin allowed a drop of vaccine to penetrate and proved more efficient for rapid vaccinations than the usual individual needle pricking. That technique, applied to person after person without sterilization of the chisel, would be intolerable nowadays, of course, but equipment sterilization then did not reflect knowledge acquired in recent decades concerning hepatitis and other conditions caused by transmissible, blood-borne viruses. Intense and wide-spread public concern accompanied the relatively small outbreaks of smallpox in the United States during the mid-century period when people recalled the devastation the disease had caused in earlier times.

Decades of diligent work throughout the world led finally to mankind's greatest disease control achievement—the eradication of smallpox. The American textbook, *Preventive Medicine and Public Health,* celebrated it in public health's typically low-key style with two contrasting sentences. In the tenth edition (1973), edited by Philip Sartwell, the sentence reads, "Smallpox *is* (italics mine) an acute exanthematous disease caused by variola virus"; and in the eleventh edition (1980), edited by John Last, it reads, "Smallpox was an acute exanthematous disease caused by variola virus." The latter is to me probably the most exciting sentence in the whole of public health literature.

Thus, before being permitted to develop a chronic disease control program I was diverted during much of 1946 to participate in three communicable disease episodes involving encephalitis, poliomyelitis, and smallpox. Each provided a learning experience, and all together they seemed a small price to pay for the opportunity that Dyar offered.

Before initiating a chronic disease control program for California I visited several eastern states where some health departments had already undertaken such efforts. These included Massachusetts, where Herbert Lombard had begun a cancer control program "with or without the cooperation [of] . . . local physicians," as the state's legislation specified to reflect determination to proceed against a growing public health problem even over potent political resistance from organized medicine. Those few official words from Massachusetts encouraged me and probably others in public health to develop necessary health programs despite opposition from powerful but relatively narrow interest groups such as medicine. My propensity to struggle on a wide front in that regard, however, provoked Halverson once to advise me, "Lester, you have to divide your fights." He taught me that you can't battle everybody at once and that some opposing parties in public health can become strong allies in other situations.

Within four years of his flatly rejecting the idea that public health should move into the chronic disease field Halverson co-authored with Malcolm Merrill, his Deputy Director, and me, "Chronic disease—the chronic disease study of the California Department of Public Health" (Halverson, Merrill, & Breslow, 1949). Presenting that paper at the annual meeting of the American Public Health Association reflected his newly acquired recognition that public health did include chronic disease control.

THE CANCER REGISTRY

Following the leads that Massachusetts and Connecticut had established, we decided to start the California chronic disease control program with a tumor (really a cancer) registry. The term "tumor registry" rather than cancer registry appealed to us because the idea conveyed by the word "cancer" was then still too frightening; physicians often didn't even tell patients that they had cancer. The Registry was to serve as a basis for formulating control efforts, in particular to determine what kinds of cancer were affecting what segments of the population and to ascertain the course of the disease among those stricken. It seemed important to know the proportion of cases that were being diagnosed in early, medium, and advanced stages of the disease, and the proportion of each that were surviving for five years, which was then the major goal of treatment. We held the conviction that health departments should contribute their expertise in health statistics and other fields toward sharing responsibility for cancer control with the medical profession and the pertinent voluntary health organization, the American Cancer Society.

Because reporting cancer cases to the state public health agency was such a new and possibly threatening venture, Halverson required me to obtain two important approvals before starting the Registry. One had to come from the California State Board of Health, a body appointed by the Governor with statutory authority to adopt regulations and policies concerning public health. Immediately after my presenting the Tumor Registry proposal to that Board one prominent member inquired, "Doctor, if we appointed you to be fire chief in our town would your first step be to count all the fires?" That difficult question aroused temporary consternation on my part; however, the Board did approve establishing the Registry.

Obtaining the second approval was more difficult. The California Medical Association's Cancer Commission, a body of prominent California physicians in important cancer-related specialties—pathology, surgery, and radiology—would have to endorse the project. The Commission invited me to present the matter at a dinner meeting in San Francisco's famed Jack's Restaurant. On the street corner en route to the restaurant meeting I noticed a newspaper headline announcing that Governor Earl Warren had introduced his state health insurance bill. (That day in late spring 1947 I did not anticipate that Governor Warren would later call upon me through Halverson to write documents and draft speeches to support his effort to achieve state health insurance.) The Governor's proposal made the Cancer Commission members, reflecting organized medicine's views, absolutely furious. Their rage, directed at me when I arrived at the restaurant, arose from the irrational assumption that the Tumor Registry was somehow connected with the Governor's "terrible idea," specifically, that he wanted the cancer cases reported so that "state doctors" could take over their care. We, of course, wanted the Registry merely to ascertain what kinds of people were being affected by what kinds of cancer and how they were faring; the notion that "state doctors" would treat the cases reported to the Registry was ludicrous. The Commission members, however, were so angered against Governor Warren's health care bill that they would not hear of the proposed Tumor Registry. Realizing that my presence was just upsetting everyone's appetite I left before dinner. The Chairman of the Cancer Commission, however, accompanied me to the door and putting his arm around my shoulder said, "Don't worry, Lester, that bill isn't going anywhere," and he advised that in a few months the difficulty would subside and the Cancer Commission would invite me back.

His prediction proved correct, and we were able to start the Tumor Registry during the latter part of 1947 on a pilot basis in nine hospitals scattered through the state—some county, some voluntary, and some university hospitals. The Registry yielded useful information about cancer and helped guide efforts toward its control, along with similar enterprises throughout the country. In California, despite the idea's first reception, it quickly gained active support from the Cancer Commission, whose members strongly encouraged participation by hospitals with which they were affiliated. By 1950 thirty-seven hospitals were participating in the Registry, including all except one of the teaching hospitals and almost half of all hospitals in the state with more than fifty beds. *California Medicine*, the official journal of the California Medical Association, accepted a paper presenting the data concerning 70,000 reported cases (Breslow, Ellis, Eaton, & Kleinman, 1951). Additional hospitals joined the Registry, and when it covered the entire San Francisco Bay Area population it became an element of the National Cancer Institute's Surveillance, Epidemiology and End Results (SEER) program in the national cancer statistical system. The Registry evolved to the point that in 1985 the State Legislature mandated statewide reporting.

Each year now the California Cancer Registry (the term cancer became acceptable to use for the Registry about 1970) adds more than 120,000 new cases to its database and its staff members respond to hundreds of inquiries about the status of cancer in the State. Since 1988 nearly 200 research projects utilizing the Registry have been initiated and almost 300 articles based on Registry data have appeared in the scientific literature. Although it is now recognized as serving a useful purpose, it was necessary originally to persuade people that public health includes responsibility for cancer data along with information about the communicable diseases. Now such information is presented in routine national reports from the SEER program in which the California data are the largest component.

One might think it ironic, considering cancer's importance as a health problem, that it took forty years after an inauspicious beginning for the Registry to reach maturity. Although some physicians, especially those concerned with cancer, soon appreciated its value, the vast majority of the profession did not. In fact, they hardly knew that the Registry existed. Most public health professionals continued to regard cancer control as far outside their mainstream and gave it little or no attention. In view of such professional apathy the California Legislature cannot be blamed for appropriating huge sums over the years to pay the technology, hospital, and medical costs of treating cancer patients, but delaying so long in taking action to ascertain who among all the state's people were developing cancer (and possibly why) and how they were faring with the disease.

CHRONIC DISEASE EPIDEMIOLOGY

Heart Disease

The late 1940s and early 1950s presented many other exhilarating days for those seeking to develop a public health approach to the chronic diseases. Supporting that trend, funds that Congress appropriated for heart disease control permitted extension somewhat more broadly into that field. Heart disease had become the nation's number one killer, and Ancel Keys was reporting from his world-wide observations the association between excessive fat consumption and coronary artery disease, the major fatal heart ailment (Keys, 1980). In the 1940s, John Gofman at the University of California, Berkeley, had identified a particular cholesterol fraction that he categorized by its weight and named SF10-20 as particularly important in generating atherosclerosis. Only years later did the relative amounts of so-called high-density and low-density blood cholesterol gain general recognition as significant in the pathogenesis of atherosclerosis. Gofman's discovery was neglected at the time evidently because it was just another new finding which did not seem to offer a path to action. Many scientific discoveries thus remain neglected because they do not fit into the paradigm of thinking that was operating when they were made.

Two cardiologists at Mt. Zion Hospital in San Francisco, Michael Friedman and Ray Rosenman, were espousing the notion that what they termed Type A (the more aggressive) personality played an important role in coronary heart disease (Rosenman & Friedman, 1975). During their early endeavors a young colleague of mine, Robert Buechley, accompanied me on a visit to Friedman. The latter received us graciously and rather early in the conversation pointed to me as a Type B personality, in Friedman's mind the desirable type because he regarded it as protective against coronary heart disease. As the conversation progressed and raised challenging questions, Friedman became increasingly irritated, in fact so agitated at what he apparently regarded as provocation that we departed early. As we walked down the hallway he was still haranguing us from his office door and finally exclaimed, "Breslow, I said you were a Type B personality, but you're damn near a Type A!" That allegation of vulnerability, especially considering the circumstances, neither caused me much worry nor attracted me to the Personality Type A–B hypothesis.

J. N. Morris, a British epidemiologist, found that London bus drivers experienced much higher coronary heart disease death rates than the conductors who had to move constantly up and down the two-decker vehicles, and from that information he suggested that physical exertion was protective against the disease (Morris & Crawford, 1958). Increasingly large-scale epidemiological studies were undertaken to ascertain what was causing the coronary heart disease epidemic. Over the years British and American investigations disclosed four major factors: high blood pressure, high blood cholesterol and especially its low density form (LDL), cigarette smoking, and physical indolence.

The large-scale epidemiological effort directed at the lung cancer epidemic in the late 1940s and 1950s attracted little public attention until the results appeared. Biomedical researchers, who had by then commandeered the National Institute of Health, insisted generally that overcoming disease required elucidating the specific pathogenic agents, their mechanisms, and then developing interventions that would block them. Controlling communicable disease had pioneered that way by discovering microbes and then immunizing people against them and/ or destroying the disease agents with antibiotics. Even though neither cancer nor the other major chronic diseases appeared to be caused by microbes, the path to control was to find the disease's biologic mechanism and then develop the "magic bullet." That concept gained tremendous support and its profound impact continues to the present time. It has not only largely taken over the National Institutes of Health as a research enterprise, but it has strongly influenced medical education in the United States.

Tom McKeown, a British epidemiologist, subsequently demonstrated the fallacy of relying so heavily on the mechanistic approach to disease control. He noted that discovering the tubercle bacillus and subsequent chemical treatment for that specific pathogenic organism had practically no effect in defeating the former "Captain of the Men of Death" (McKeown, 1976). He properly attributed the massive historic decline in tuberculosis overwhelmingly to improved general living standards— better food, housing, and working conditions. Introducing drugs that restrained the tubercle bacillus came later and made scarcely a blip in the story of how tuberculosis has been defeated over the years. True, a biologic mechanism is involved, but knowing that mechanism and acting on it did not significantly affect the centuries-long struggle against tuberculosis. Specific control of the disease mechanism by antibiotic therapy applied to the invading microbic agent has only slightly facilitated the decline in recent decades. Social conditions have been the principal long-term influence on tuberculosis.

The notion that the twentieth-century, noncommunicable, chronic disease epidemics such as coronary heart disease and lung cancer are also essentially biosocial phenomena came forcibly to me while visiting Yugoslavia in the late 1950s. Traveling in order to become acquainted with colleagues in other countries and to compare findings at meetings had become an integral part of the developing chronic disease control enterprise. While I was visiting a hospital in Belgrade, my hosts showed me various patients and then obviously expected me to ask some questions. To one query, "Do you have any coronary heart disease cases?" the prompt response was to show me several such patients. To my next question, "Who gets coronary heart disease here?" the physician took my hand, drew his fingers across my palm, and smiled as he replied, "Men who have smooth hands like yours: artists, merchants, professors, writers, people of that sort—not hard-working people."

That answer propelled me into thinking about the trend of coronary heart disease. It opened my eyes to the fact that as parts of the world become more industrialized and commercialized, that highly fatal condition appears earliest among the more affluent people living there, those who lead softer lives. At first it rarely occurs among those people who work hard physically. Then as more and more people in industrialized society are able to avoid performing physically demanding labor and have more income so that they can eat more fat and smoke cigarettes, coronary heart disease affects them, too.

I recalled that our 1930s medical school professors taught us that a typical heart attack patient (myocardial infarction, the often fatal consequence of coronary heart disease) was a fat banker who wore a gold chain across his vest. The disease did not frequently affect ordinary, hardworking Americans. Two decades later, myocardial infarction occurred commonly in the United States Caucasian male population, but still not among African-American males. The latter group, as well as some people in developing countries, later encountered these same, relatively more affluent living conditions, and they have recently been suffering the consequent disease more frequently than other people who encountered such conditions in earlier years. An American Epidemiological Society meeting in the mid-twentieth century featured a debate on whether black men had a racial immunity to coronary heart disease because it then occurred so rarely among them. Thereafter, the disease increased among African-American men, at first young ones, and then up the age scale. By the 1990s their coronary heart disease mortality rate exceeded that among Caucasian men up to age 65. Further support for the scenario arose in my mind during a 1983 visit to the Papua New Guinea highlands. Some local hospital nurses there answered my query, "Who gets coronary heart disease here?" by replying "the Aussies." (The Australians had for some time occupied Papua New Guinea where they lived a more affluent lifestyle than the natives.) When I persisted, "Do any Papuans get it?" they responded, "Only a very few men," and to "What kind of Papuans," the answer was, "Those who deal in money."

Epidemic coronary heart disease thus begins at the top of the social ladder and proceeds downward. The disease occurrence also declines first at the top as more affluent and better educated people learn to avoid the major risk factors. Like the other major chronic diseases, its epidemic course extends over decades rather than the weeks or months characteristic of the acute communicable disease epidemics. The chronic disease epidemic has been a twentieth-century phenomenon, now unfortunately extending into the twenty-first century when and wherever in the world beginning affluence encourages living patterns that impose a burden on the coronary arteries that exceeds their biological competence. We are simply not genetically constructed to withstand so much fatty food, physical indolence, cigarette smoke, and the situations that provoke high blood pressure. Coronary heart disease is thus a classic biosocial event. Regrettably, the psychosocially generated habits seem attractive because they yield such pleasures as the taste of fats and nicotine's psychological effects. Acquiring them is easy and giving them up is difficult. The so-called Western lifestyle is fortunately declining in those countries where it originated, with a consequent decline in coronary heart disease, but unfortunately that lifestyle is now spreading into developing countries and the epidemic is now ascending there. Policies of some Western countries accelerate and enlarge the adverse consequences in those newly affected countries, for example, by encouraging cigarette sales there (and thereby enriching tobacco companies located in "advanced" nations where sales are declining).

Lung Cancer

Lung cancer is similar to coronary heart disease in following a socially determined path. The disease was extremely rare in 1900, grew to prominence during the twentieth century in the so-called developed world, and only at the start of the twenty-first century is it increasing rapidly in the developing world while declining in countries where it started.

Thus, the two major modern epidemics, lung cancer and coronary heart disease, have not only certain biological characteristics but also definite social origins. The circumstances in which people live (e.g., the availability and marketing of manufactured cigarettes and fatty foods, the lack of physical demands, and the way people respond to these conditions) have obviously kindled those epidemics.

Like other people, epidemiologists do not readily escape the influence of their current social situations. Not many epidemiologists nowadays have actively joined the struggle against tobacco and other causes of disease; although there are exceptions, most regard that struggle as "someone else's business." Such an attitude differentiates epidemiologists at the turn of the current century from those typically involved in the late 1940s and 1950s who saw the field mainly as a way to advance health, not merely as another science to pursue. For example, Richard Doll and John Pemberton joined the hunger marches of the unemployed in the 1930s as students. Doll not only played a leading role in finding cigarette smoke to be a cause of lung cancer and other diseases, but he has strongly participated in the struggle against tobacco by testifying in legal actions; Pemberton became an activist against malnutrition as well as investigating it scientifically; Jeremiah Morris joined with Pemberton in organizing a Socialist Study Club that had to be renamed the Hippocratic Club to avoid its being banned for political activity.

Although in the Bureau of Chronic Disease we focused much early control effort on lung cancer and coronary heart disease epidemiology, we also devoted attention to other ways of attacking the chronic disease problems. For example, the Pap test that would detect cervical cancer early and thus make cure possible was not being widely applied, mainly because pathologists maintained that only they could examine the test slides for microscopic evidence of the disease or its precursors. They insisted that not even specially trained technicians could screen the slides and refer suspect cases to pathologists, who would make the definitive determinations. With that professional stranglehold on the technique, the Pap test would have little public health benefit. Only wealthy people would be able to pay a pathologist to examine the slides, whereas our studies and others showed that the disease affected poor women much more frequently than the affluent. With the treatment for cervical cancer available even then, the disease could have been largely controlled. Instead, during the 25 years after 1945 an average of more than 10,000 women in the United States died annually from cervical cancer—250,000 altogether. Public health agencies generally failed to incorporate the Pap screening test into their programs, and the NCI and the CDC did practically nothing to advance its use. During the subsequent 25 years (1970–1995) more than 125,000 additional women died from the disease, largely unnecessarily. Although sharply declining as a cause of death in recent years, cervical cancer has resulted in about 400,000 deaths in the past half-century and is still responsible for more than 4,000 death each year. Experience with cervical cancer has been a major public health failure. By the turn of the century affluent and well-educated women had been largely freed of the disease, but older, poor, and less educated women, especially those from Latin America, remain quite vulnerable to morbidity and mortality from it. Enthusiasm is mounting again for use of the Pap smear, a half-century after the technology became available.

In California we devoted some of the federally available cancer funds to train a few pathologists in the technique, hoping that they would ultimately organize efficient services with technicians screening the slides under professional supervision. More aggressive, however, and determined to extend the Pap test use promptly, a San Diego gynecological group would not wait for the pathologists. They first mastered examining slides themselves and then trained their own technicians to screen them. Only gradually did further technician training bring the Pap smear into substantial use. Unfortunately, thousands of cervical cancer deaths still occur annually among poor, uneducated, older women who never received a Pap smear or even heard of it. This disgraceful aspect of American medical service is seldom noted even more than fifty years after the demonstration of the Pap smear's effectiveness in identifying cervical cancer cases early enough for cure.

Multiphasic Screening

Technology for early detection of several chronic diseases was being increasingly developed and used in the late 1940s. The chest x-ray had already become prominent in tuberculosis case-finding, routine medical examinations usually included blood pressure measurement for identifying previously unknown hypertension, and automated methods were just becoming available for determining blood sugar levels and thus finding diabetes early in asymptomatic persons. These advances emphasized the significance of applied medical research that could lead to useful technology for public health.

At that time each group of professional and lay people concerned with minimizing the toll from a particular chronic disease such as cancer, tuberculosis, or diabetes included in their strategy a single-disease screening technology that would disclose cases of "their" disease early and thus in the most treatable stage. Reflecting on that fact led me to propose a more efficient method of dealing with the chronic diseases as a whole. The greatest expense in screening for particular diseases was assembling and keeping records on the people who would participate. The Tuberculosis Association would provide chest x-rays to one group of people, while the Heart Association was promoting blood pressure determination to others. The Diabetes Association would soon be encouraging mass blood-sugar testing with the newly available automated methods, and the Cancer Society was already trying to popularize the Pap smear among women.

Combining such screening examinations into a single program with unified promotion and record systems seemed an obvious next step for chronic disease control (Breslow, 1950). Thus the concept of multiphasic screening (i.e., the examination of a large number of people with a whole series of tests for detecting several disease processes in a single operation) emerged. The term "multiphasic" jumped into my mind during preparation for such a screening project among San Jose cannery workers (Canelo, Bissell, Abrams, & Breslow, 1949). As we were planning that endeavor I recalled the term "multiphasic" from the Minnesota Multiphasic Personality Inventory (MMPI), which had been developed at the University of Minnesota in the 1930s while I was a student there. The term seemed well suited for this new chronic disease control venture.

In carrying out the first multiphasic screening project we selected San Jose cannery workers as the pilot group. The local health department and county medical society co-sponsored the event in which 945 cannery workers were screened with miniature chest x-ray films, blood specimens, and urine samples, as well as personal and medical history forms in order to detect the possible presence of pulmonary disease, heart disease, syphilis, diabetes, and kidney disease. During that project we encountered some fascinating logistic and technological problems; for example, the available automated determination of blood sugar level involved dripping some chemicals into a test tube, adding a small amount of the participant's blood, and then attaching the test tube into position on a rack that a ten-foot-long machine then moved around to stations at thirty-second intervals. At each of the several stations on the machine's path additional chemicals would be added, and at a certain point on the route the test tube contents were heated and then cooled. The cooling required moving the test tubes through a vessel of water kept cold by manually adding ice; keeping sufficient ice in the water to maintain adequate coldness became a significant logistic difficulty for us in the first multiphasic screening. Such was medical technology fifty years ago. After the San Jose experience we carried out several successful demonstrations of multiphasic screening in other California communities. Though the term is no longer widely used, the idea of a series of well-established tests in routine medical check-ups continues.

Illustrating how public health ideas and approaches to problems spread, shortly after we published an account of our multiphasic screening experience in San Jose, I was approached by two staff members of the International Longshore and Warehouse Men's Union (ILWU)-Pacific Maritime Association (PMA) Health and Welfare Fund. They came with a problem arising from a medical services contract that the ILWU-PMA fund had negotiated with the Kaiser-Permanente Health Plan, which was just then getting underway in the San Francisco Bay Area. The contract, a big step in those days for the fledgling Kaiser prepaid health plan, specifically included periodic physical examinations for the approximately 6,000 longshore union members. When the ILWU-PMA staff members approached the Kaiser-Permanente physicians to arrange those physical examinations, they were told that they should send the men over. The physicians did not believe that longshoremen would actually come for such examinations, and hence had been willing to put the item into the contract. The ILWU-PMA staff repeatedly requested the Kaiser-Permanente doctors to specify how they wanted to handle the examinations, and each time were told to simply send them over. When the ILWU-PMA staff informed the doctors that groups of twenty, forty, or sixty men would come, and asked how many groups they wanted at a time, the doctors still replied that they didn't expect the men to come. They did not understand that the union organized longshore work, assigning twenty men each to gangs that unload or load a ship in 10–20 hours. During the following few days during their rest period gangs would be dispatched for examinations. Any gang members failing to report for examination would go to the bottom of the list and have to wait longer for another job. The union really did control its members' work schedules. The Kaiser-Permanente medical group finally realized that actually performing 6,000 physical examinations as required by the contract would overwhelm their still-limited resources and requested time to consider the matter.

Meanwhile, the ILWU-PMA staff came to us inquiring whether multiphasic screening, which they had read about, might not solve the problem. I responded that it would disclose important health abnormalities early and inexpensively, as intended by periodic health examinations. They then asked me to "sell" the idea to Kaiser-Permanente. I demurred and insisted that the ILWU-PMA staff would have to do any "selling"; I was not inclined to tell physicians how they should do their work. Subsequently the Kaiser-Permanente doctors visited us to explore the possibility of multiphasic screening as a solution to the matter. I ultimately entered into a rather interesting conference on the issue with the Permanente Medical Director, Dr. E. Richard Weinerman; Dr. Sidney Garfield, the Permanente Medical Group's founder; the "Old Man," Henry J. Kaiser; and Harry Bridges, head of the ILWU. Bridges was the only one who showed cold feet; he expressed great concern about ordering longshoremen into such a newfangled checkup. He proposed that we first send a postal card to each man inquiring whether he would accept the multiphasic examination in lieu of a regular physician's checkup. We objected to that procedure, asserting that what a man wrote or didn't write in response would not reliably indicate the idea's acceptability. Acceding to that judgment, Bridges then demanded that Weinerman and I explain the plan at a union meeting. We agreed and a few days later went to the San Francisco Auditorium where all 6,000 union members came for a regular meeting. Astonished at the full attendance, I inquired about it and was told that each man was checked off entering the auditorium through one of several doors assigned alphabetically by name for him to enter. If not checked off he was fined $25, which constituted a considerable amount in those days. What happened if a man was hospitalized with a broken leg or stayed at the bedside of his dying mother? The answer: "That would just cost $25." There were no excuses for not participating in meetings of that union-enforced democracy.

It was my first encounter with meeting hall microphones, six of them down two aisles. Dozens of men lined up quietly behind the microphones after Dick Weinerman and I had made our presentations. They were each allowed a brief period to ask a question or say whatever they wanted, damn the government, insist on "regular doctor examinations," criticize Bridges, or anything else. Bridges sat way back on the platform, letting Dick and me take considerable verbal pummeling at the rostrum. After considerable discussion, however, the members overwhelmingly approved proceeding with the multiphasic screening as the "checkup."

Based on favorable experience with the longshoremen, the Kaiser-Permanente Medical Group incorporated multiphasic screening into the Health Plan's routine services. By 1970 the Group was performing 50,000 such examinations on Kaiser Health Plan members annually, evidently because they readily accepted them and the Kaiser physicians looked upon multiphasic screening as an efficient way of responding to patients' growing desires for periodic health checkups (Collen, 1978). Their popularity expanded as more people began to realize their potential for disclosing early stages of particular diseases when treatment can be most effective. What the Kaiser Health Plan physicians called automated multiphasic health testing has continued in various forms, usually with a small sample of venous blood such as in the now commonly used blood profile (i.e., ascertaining hemoglobin level, the proportion of various types of blood cells, cholesterol, sugar, and other blood constituents), the results of which provide clues to several diseases.

The multiphasic screening experience also prompted me to develop the concept of secondary prevention (Breslow, 1956a). Recognizing the need for attention to the chronic disease problem, the American Medical

Association, American Hospital Association, American Public Health Association, and the American Public Welfare Association, following their 1947 joint statement on chronic illness, formed the Commission on Chronic Illness in 1949. The 1947 statement had dealt largely with diagnosis, treatment, rehabilitation, long-term care, and other means of handling the chronic illness problem. I was given responsibility as a Commission member for leading its chronic disease prevention work. In that capacity I proposed that chronic disease prevention can take two forms: (1) primary prevention (i.e., the avoidance of disease occurrence, as by not smoking cigarettes), and (2) secondary prevention (i.e., detecting disease early in its course and intervening to avoid adverse consequences, for example, by taking the blood pressure of asymptomatic persons and sometimes discovering hypertension and with treatment minimizing the risk of heart and kidney damage). Volume I of the Commission's report defines primary prevention as "averting the occurrence of disease" and secondary prevention as "halting the progression of a disease from its early unrecognized state to a more severe one and preventing complications or sequelae of disease" (Commission on Chronic Illness, 1957a, p. 16). The notion of secondary prevention has promoted the related concept of health monitoring, that is, periodic examinations for systematically detecting early signs of disease and its precursors.

OTHER DIRECTIONS IN CHRONIC DISEASE CONTROL

Besides epidemiological studies of chronic disease leading to primary prevention, the development of multiphasic screening, and the concept of secondary prevention, our chronic disease control work took other directions. We explored several approaches to the problem, including rehabilitation, nutrition, and nursing home care. Mainly, however, we concentrated on controlling major fatal diseases such as cancer and heart disease with primary and secondary prevention.

Even though cancer therapy was becoming more effective in the 1940s than it had been previously, people still largely regarded it as a dread disease for which conventional measures offered little hope. The field was ripe for "miracle cures" and unscrupulous people took lucrative advantage of the situation. The American Cancer Society's California Division and Bureau of Chronic Disease efforts toward legislative passage of a strong cancer quackery law bore fruit only after ten years, when such a law was finally adopted in 1959. A statutory Cancer Advisory Council then advised the Bureau's Cancer Diagnosis and Therapy Evaluation Unit in administering the law, which resulted over the next decade in banning six useless cancer remedies and two diagnostic tests that were being commonly used to prey on gullible Californians with such names as Hoxsey, Laetrile, Koch, and Krebiozen. Cease and desist orders had been issued against twenty-three individuals and criminal charges filed against seventeen of them by 1969.

The American Cancer Society invited me to lead a small group of epidemiologists to examine a Canadian surgeon's claims that simple mastectomy was as effective in breast cancer treatment as the traditional Halsted operation, which was a comprehensive and often mutilating removal of the breast, axillary nodes, and adjacent tissue in cases of breast cancer. Our group was asked in company with several surgeons, pathologists, and radiologists selected by the American Cancer Society to review the evidence for the Halsted procedure's greater effectiveness than a simpler operation. Finding essentially no published literature supporting the radical mastectomy, we inquired before the conference whether our colleagues from the cancer-related clinical specialties had other data to support using the Halsted operation. They presented none. A leading surgeon of the time had developed the procedure, and it simply became accepted. When we pointed to the lack of evidence for the procedure, the cancer treatment specialists became upset and the meeting broke up in confusion. Our clinical colleagues would not even consider the challenge from the Canadian surgeon or our views; they knew what to do about breast cancer. That experience taught me once again the power of medical orthodoxy and the need for evidence-based medicine. It took years for U.S. surgeons to accept simple mastectomy, and more recently lumpectomy, together with radiation and chemotherapy as a means of treating the disease. The Halsted operation has become virtually a matter of history. Over the past few decades medical decision making has generally turned away from heavy dependence on prevailing professional opinion toward greater reliance on health services research, such as the clinical trial our British epidemiologic colleague, Archie Cochrane, advocated, which has fortunately become prominent in recent years (Bosch, 2003).

During the late 1940s and early 1950s enthusiasm for addressing chronic (noncommunicable) disease gradually expanded in public health circles. I was fortunate enough to be active in that period, serving, for example, as founding Chairman of the American Public Health Association Committee on Chronic Diseases and Rehabilitation, as President of the Public Health Cancer Association, and later of the Association of State Chronic Disease Program Directors.

As further evidence of public health's advance into the chronic disease arena, in 1950 the California Conference of Local Health Officers adopted a guide, the Chronic Disease Control Program in Local Health Departments. By 1953 the Conference had asked the State Department of Public Health to survey local activities in the field as a basis for further action. Subsequently, the American Public Health Association issued a similar publication for the national effort.

In 1950 Kenneth Maxcy, then editing the classic American textbook *Preventive Medicine and Hygiene,* initiated by Milton Rosenau in 1914 and more recently titled *Public Health and Preventive Medicine,* asked me to write a chapter in that text's seventh edition on what he proposed be called "Diseases of Senescence." Because of my objection to characterizing them so dishearteningly but Maxcy's insistence on that term, we compromised on "Senescence, Chronic Disease, and Disability in Adults." I took care early in the chapter to differentiate the process of aging from those pathologic processes that often accompany aging and eventuate in the chronic diseases (Breslow, 1951). Only in the ninth (1965) edition, however, when Phillip Sartwell had taken over the editorship, was the term "senescence" removed from the chapter's title. Also at that time, Sartwell began expanding his attention to the chronic disease field, including, for example, a separate chapter on cancer authored by Abraham Lilienfeld (Sartwell, 1965).

Interest within the California Legislature led to passing Assembly Concurrent Resolution No. 42 in 1947 requesting the Department "to investigate the problems involved in the reduction of deaths and disability from cancer and other chronic diseases . . . and report to the 1949 session of the Legislature." The report's recommendations for state financing of a concerted, coordinated attack on the problems came to naught in 1949 and again in 1951. Meanwhile federal support kept the Bureau's program going. It was not until 1955 that the California Legislature finally appropriated funds for support of our efforts, and then only for two specific endeavors: study of smog and alcoholism. By 1960, however, the California Chronic Disease Program had achieved sufficient national attention to be awarded a Lasker Award "in recognition of a concept, an organization and a public health physician."

ADVANCES IN CHRONIC DISEASE CONTROL

Chronic disease control work as an aspect of public health was becoming reasonably respectable by the 1960s. The Commission on Chronic Illness report, initiation of American Public Health Association activity in the field, growing state health department programs, and vigorous epidemiological research endeavors reflected increasing professional acceptance of the idea. As yet, of course, the chronic disease toll was still high. Heart disease mortality rates had continued their upward trend until the 1950s, and cancer even longer (among other reasons because the lung cancer epidemic was erupting among women). It was hardly the time to declare victory; we seemed actually to be losing the battle.

During the last quarter of the twentieth century, however, the tide definitely turned. Heart disease and stroke deaths had been declining steadily and sharply since mid-century, and cancer mortality as a whole turned downward in the 1990s; in fact, cancer mortality had begun declining among children as early as the 1950s and subsequently at older ages. Although disability from chronic disease still imposes a heavy population burden the chronic disease epidemic is clearly receding. Evidence may be seen in Table 3, which indicates the chronic disease mortality trend in the United States during the latter half of the twentieth century. Three major forms of chronic disease—heart disease, cerebrovascular disease, and cancer—dominated the pattern of death during most of the last century. This epidemic ascendancy and then decline have been as noteworthy as the control of communicable disease, which has extended over several centuries. Coronary (ischemic) heart disease, whose major manifestation—myocardial infarction (heart attack)—which occurred only rarely during the early part of the century, reached a peak several decades ago and is now falling rapidly. Cancer mortality as a whole kept rising due to lung cancer until the 1990s, but even lung cancer is now declining.

Although advances in medical practice for individuals have played an important role in chronic disease control, efforts directed toward the population as a whole (e.g., educational and screening campaigns) have made highly significant contributions. Development and implementation

TABLE 3 Age-Adjusted Death Rates for Selected Causes of Death, United States 1950–1997

	1950	1960	1970	1980	1990	1997
All causes	842	761	714	586	520	479
Heart diseases	307	286	254	202	152	131
Ischemic heart disease	—	—	—	150	103	83
Cerebrovascular disease	89	80	66	41	28	26
Cancer	125	126	130	131	135	126
Respiratory system	13	19	28	36	41	39
All other cancer	112	107	102	95	94	87

Source: National Center for Health Statistics. Health, United States, 1999. Hyattsville MD. 1999.

of steps to reduce smoking and high blood pressure illustrate how influencing people's behavior has facilitated chronic disease control.

Terris (1983) has described disease control during the twentieth century as the first and second epidemiologic revolutions: the first against the communicable diseases and the second against the noncommunicable (chronic) diseases. That is certainly an accurate depiction. Although neither "revolution" has completed its tasks, the first has reduced communicable disease mortality to a small fraction of its impact in 1900, and the second (which has been underway only during the second half of the century) has curtailed mortality from the major chronic diseases by more than 50 percent of their rate in 1950. Disease control progress has yielded probably the greatest health improvement, at least that manifested by increased longevity, in the history of mankind: an extension of life from 47 to 77 years or 66 percent during one century.

A Larger View of Public Health 5

During World War II, almost all agencies and institutions in the United States, including those concerned with public health, largely committed themselves to the war effort. Only after the war could they consider how to reorient their organizations and activities to the rapidly changing social circumstances that were challenging public health and other social enterprises at mid-century.

It was obvious that new health problems had arisen and that public health must adapt itself to dealing with them. Tuberculosis still played a considerable role and poliomyelitis, smallpox, and other communicable disease outbreaks were occurring from time to time, but health interest was shifting to the noncommunicable conditions such as heart disease, cancer, and stroke, which were then causing most of the morbidity and mortality. How public health should approach these matters began to receive consideration, as the previous chapter has indicated.

The new health situation reflected both the aging of the population and the way people lived. From 1900 to 1950 the proportion of persons over age 65 had increased more than 50 percent; life expectancy (fifty-fifty chance of number of years to be lived from birth) had risen from 47 years in 1900 to 68 in 1950. The fact that people were extending life into later decades mainly reflected escaping high mortality in their earlier years, but they were now encountering biological damage in the form of chronic diseases resulting from various factors that had been in play during their longer years of life. In the 1940s we were not much aware of the specific causes of that damage, but such knowledge was accumulating. We now realize that vast changes had been occurring, not only in the aging of the population but also in the ways people were living. Industrial employment had boomed during the first half of the century,

69

and women had entered the war industries extensively in the late 1930s and 1940s. The forklift and other technological advances had lessened physical demands at work; less physical exertion and more calories, especially from fats, were available to larger numbers of people; and cigarette marketing became highly successful. A new style of life, which we have come to realize induced the chronic disease epidemic, had become the norm.

Seeking to advance health in this new era gradually led to the perception that public health included three major arms for dealing with disease. A rational and comprehensive approach to public health's mission—later expressed in the 1988 Institute of Medicine statement assuring "conditions in which people can be healthy" (p. 7)—requires attention to all three ways whereby the mission can be accomplished: (1) assuring access to good quality personal health services, (2) environmental control measures, and (3) providing a milieu that encourages healthful personal behavior (Institute of Medicine, 1988). Meanwhile medical science and its applications have yielded some spectacular achievements, and thus encouraged the tendency to attribute health advances almost totally to medicine. Although personal health services are highly important, and thus public health must address them, the other two ways of protecting and advancing health (i.e., environmental measures and influencing behavior) also require substantial attention. Table 4 illustrates this concept.

Personal Health Services

How to provide medical services was gaining prominence as a health issue in the United States at the middle of the century. Progress in medical science and the correspondingly improved education of physicians were yielding better surgical care, antibiotic treatment of microbic diseases, cancer chemotherapy, and other increasingly effective services, along with greater medical specialization. These rapid developments resulted in significant advances in America's medical services and popular expectation that a cure would be found for every major condition. A widespread feeling arose that, simply, the more funds for medical research the more quickly the cures would appear.

Growth in the medical profession's size and competence and the Hill-Burton program, which allocated federal funds for hospital construction, however, did not bring the remarkable health benefits of better medical services to all Americans. Millions of them, who were socially disadvantaged by race-ethnicity and/or income level, had been shunted into

TABLE 4 Means of Reducing Mortality and Morbidity from Selected Common Conditions

Condition	Behavioral influences	Environmental measures	Personal health care
Automobile trauma	Driver training Avoid driving while under the influence of alcohol or other drugs	Highway construction Automobile construction	Ambulance service Emergency medical care Rehabilitation care
Dental caries	Prudent diet Brush teeth	Fluoridation Reduce production and promotion of refined carbohydrates	Dental care
Myocardial infarction	Increase exercise Prudent diet Stop cigarette smoking	Alter food supply to reduce intake of foods that raise blood cholesterol level	Screen for risk factors and attend to them Ambulance service Coronary care units
Lung cancer	Stop cigarette smoking	Reduce production and promotion of cigarettes Reduce occupational exposures that cause lung cancer	Detect disease early and treat promptly
Infant deaths	Maintain good diet Avoid child abuse	Maintain hygiene in home Assure safe water supply	Pediatric care

Source: P. Sartwell, ed. (1973). *Preventive Medicine and Public Health* (10th ed., p. 634). New York: Appleton-Century-Crofts.

inferior services or sometimes denied care altogether. Even those who were fortunate enough to gain access to the mainstream system often suffered from its cost and sometimes inadequate quality.

An example of how a health department can become involved in the quality of medical and related services came several years after the introduction of the Pap smear and its commercialization. The California Department of Public Health Laboratory Services Division, in carrying out its duties for licensing and regulating medical laboratory services, discovered that some California physicians were sending their cervix smear specimens to an out-of-state laboratory in order to reduce cost. Obtaining some slides returned from the out-of-state laboratory and the corresponding reports, the Laboratory Services Division staff ascertained that the specimens had not even been stained and thus could not have been properly interpreted! That experience augmented my appreciation of the hazards that inadequate medical service can cause, and how a public health department can intervene to protect the public.

As early as the 1930s, the findings and report of the Committee on the Costs of Medical Care (CCMC), headed by Ray Lyman Wilbur, had aroused interest in these matters (Committee on the Costs of Medical Care, 1932). The CCMC report stressed the need for a comprehensive national approach to medical care services in the United States. That idea has, of course, long seemed obvious to many serious students of the issue, but politically it has proved very difficult to implement fully.

Traditional public health leaders consistently eschewed any concern or interest in general medical care services. They did so mainly to minimize tension with organized medicine, which opposed governmental participation in providing medical services and exercised considerable political power over public health, including appointment of health officers and initiation of public health programs. Some progressive health officers recognized the importance of making the increasingly effective medical services available to disadvantaged segments of society, but they had to limit how far they would go in that direction because of opposition by organized medicine's political power. Most health officers simply avoided the issue by inaction, which they justified by insisting that public health's mission did not include medical care and that venturing into it would only jeopardize what public health agencies could and should do. They stuck largely to the six basic public health functions that Haven Emerson had espoused and that the American Public Health Association had adopted in 1940: vital statistics, communicable disease control, environmental sanitation, maternal and child health services (especially for the poor), health education, and public health laboratory services. Actually, these accepted public health functions did include certain medical care services, particularly immunizations for communicable disease control and prenatal and child health care for the poor, but a stop sign usually confronted health officers approaching any more general medical care.

The latter had become a significant issue for indigents and obviously required some social action. Public welfare agencies picked up the responsibility and linked it with financial assistance to poor people. Whereas physicians in small-town America had generally been providing free medical services to the poor, the growing cities embraced large numbers of indigents residing in extensive neighborhoods and obviously made governmental participation in providing medical services to them necessary. The medical profession accepted that trend as long as it was handled as financial assistance to the poor, carried no implication of governmental direction of personal health service, and generally provided income to physicians. Welfare administrators, for whom medical service was simply another budgeted benefit for recipients, thus took charge of public medical care in which part-time physicians played some, but usually peripheral, management roles.

Failure to include medical coverage in the original Social Security Act of 1935 had been a setback usually attributed to President Roosevelt's belief that fighting for it against medical opposition would endanger achieving the other benefits he sought. I. G. Falk, Yale professor of public health and member of the American Public Health Association, and a few other like-minded public health professionals kept pressing to incorporate medical care services into public health (Falk, 1958). Another major influence came from Canadian medical care developments, which were ahead of those in the United States. Based on his experience working in the Canadian province approach to providing medical services, Fred Mott took the lead in organizing a medical care program for the United Mine Workers of America. Other unions also entered the health insurance battle, often joining with employers in establishing local health plans for their members.

Activists like Falk and Mott attracted a coterie of young physicians in the American Public Health Association who sought to stimulate the nation's public health agencies into taking appropriate responsibility for medical care services. Though their efforts were vigorously resisted by traditionalists in public health, in 1948 the American Public Health Association formed a Medical Care Section, and caught up in that movement within the American Public Health Association, during 1960–1962 I chaired its Committee on Medical Care Administration. My principal effort in that position was to stress the potential of providing public access to medical services as a means of advancing health rather than simply for economic relief. I believed that was the reason for making such services a necessary component of public health endeavor. If adequately provided in quality and quantity, medical services could substantially help safeguard health in the population and as such constituted an element of public health.

My involvement in medical care had actually started in the late 1940s when Governor Earl Warren, a liberal Republican, advocated a California state health insurance plan and asked the state health officer for assistance. Wilton Halverson, as most health officers of that time would have done, personally declined to support the proposal, but he did suggest informally to Warren that I might be helpful. Accordingly, I was quietly drafted to assist with the Governor's speeches on the topic and was careful to keep that activity away from the chronic disease program that we were developing at the time. Despite Warren's eager efforts his health insurance venture came to naught.

President's Commission on Health Needs of the Nation

Early in 1952 Dr. Russell Lee, a well-known medical innovator who had founded and directed the Palo Alto Medical Clinic, telephoned me to ask that I discuss with him an opportunity with the recently appointed President's Commission on Health Needs of the Nation. Accepting the invitation to confer on the matter as a great honor but not anticipating any further involvement, I was received in Lee's small, tidy office at the Clinic. He informed me that as a member of President Truman's Health Commission he had been delegated to recruit me as the Commission's Study Director. The Commission chairman, Paul Magnuson, had brought in someone from the Veteran's Administration to head the staff work. After a very short time, however, three Commission members—Lowell Reed, who was then Dean of the Johns Hopkins University School of Public Health; Russell Lee; and Albert J. Hayes, president of the International Association of Machinists—insisted on having me as the actual Study Director. The man originally chosen would handle administrative details, but I would be working directly with the Commission on the report itself. The task entailed leading a small staff under close Commission direction to produce the document by December 1952. Having sought unsuccessfully to obtain national health legislation Truman wished to have at least a report on what should be done "to meet the health needs of the general public [and] . . . the long-term requirements for safeguarding and improving the health of the Nation" (President's Commission on Health Needs of the Nation, 1952).

Although it was indeed an exciting opportunity, I explained to Dr. Lee why it was utterly impossible for me to accept the position. With three young children in Berkeley I did not want to spend the necessary nine or ten months in Washington, D.C., away from my family; and since the work must start immediately it would be impractical to move the family. Further, the State Department of Public Health undoubtedly would not grant me a leave for such a purpose. In addition, in public health we did not make (and did not expect to make) large incomes, and what the Commission would be able to pay would not cover my family expenses in Berkeley plus separate living costs for me while working in Washington. Finally, the Commission would be completing its most critical work during the time of the annual American Public Health Association meeting, to which I was already committed. Having written on the back of an envelope some notes about these obviously substantial reasons I must decline the position, Lee thanked me and I expressed appreciation for the consideration and returned to Berkeley.

About two weeks later he called and asked to see me a second time, saying that he still wanted to talk to me about the position. I reminded him that we had discussed the matter and, I thought, had settled it. At Lee's insistence, however, I acquiesced to the second visit which he started by telling me that my problems had been solved. First, he produced a letter from the President of the State Board of Health granting me a leave from the Department for the year. Then, remarking that he understood very well the need to attend to one's young family, he handed me about twenty-five travel requests (TRs) that could be used to obtain airline tickets. Whenever I wished to visit Berkeley to see my family I could go to the airport and use a TR to obtain a round-trip ticket to California, Lee emphasized that the Commission would understand the absences. Further, because the work would require seven days a week, the Commission would pay me for a seven-day week, extra-scale, which would enable me to maintain the family in Berkeley and keep an apartment for myself in Washington. Finally, during the annual APHA meeting week, which Lee acknowledged I surely must attend, he himself would take my desk in Washington during that critical period of the Commission's work. Lee covered all these points very matter of factly within about five minutes, checking each one off on the very envelope he had marked during the first visit. I was flabbergasted and said that I would have to talk with my wife. "That's fine," he replied, because he wanted me to accompany him to Washington the next night.

Although it would be hard on the family, after we discussed the matter, I decided to accept the position. Lee and I met at the plane, and immediately after we were airborne, he opened his briefcase and pulled out about ten legal-size handwritten pages. Stating that he had written his views on how the Commission work should proceed, he asked me to comment. Although tired from having finished necessary tasks before departing, I read his notes carefully. To his insistent questioning about what I thought of his ideas I finally responded, "Not much." He asked why and after hearing my explanation, he took back his notes and tore them up. Then he removed his shoes, loosened his tie, and fell asleep. Although he was a powerful and seemingly domineering personality, Lee's equanimity and willingness to consider another person's ideas were equally impressive.

Paul Magnuson, an orthopedic surgeon from Chicago and the Commission Chair, received me warmly in Washington. Although he would be in the office often during the ensuing months, he left the Commission's real leadership to Lowell Reed and Russell Lee, who turned the work essentially over to me under their general surveillance. I found a small apartment and learned to make simple suppers for myself following the twelve-hour work days, seven per week (with occasional half-days off) as Lee had indicated would be necessary. I learned later that some weeks after my arrival in Washington, Secret Service agents had visited Magnuson demanding that he fire me because my name appeared on a McCarthy-inspired list, in those days a powerful blacklist based on alleged revolutionary political activity. He responded that the agents should "get the hell out" of his office, that the President had asked him to run the Commission's work, and that he was going to do so. For the Commission, this apparently ended the matter of my appearing on that infamous roster.

The Commission members represented a wide range of views on health issues and taught me a great deal about advocacy and negotiating points of view. Walter Reuther, founder of the Congress of Industrial Organizations (CIO) from his base in the United Automobile Workers, and Dean Clark, who was then director of the Massachusetts General Hospital and had played a leading role in advancing progressive notions about how medical care should be organized, constituted one end of the ideological spectrum. On the other could be found Chester Barnard, an industrialist and then the chairman of the National Science Foundation; Magnuson himself; and Joseph Hinsey, Dean of the Cornell University Medical College. Their discussions were enhanced by non-professionals interested in health such as Elizabeth Magee, general secretary of the National Consumers League, and Clarence Poe, editor of the *Progressive Farmer Magazine*. In his letter transmitting the final report, Magnuson stated, "Dealing with a highly controversial subject and representing many divergent points of view in our society, they [the Commission members] nevertheless have sat around the table like good Americans and thrashed out their differences in amicable fashion. Their experience is clear proof that these issues can be discussed intelligently without resorting to misleading slogans or heated invective" (President's Commission on Health Needs of the Nation, 1952).

One must wonder why that pattern seems so abandoned today when "misleading slogans and heated invective" typically overshadow consideration of key health issues. Changes in communication technology perhaps contribute to the difference. Referring to "the indispensable aid of a highly competent staff," Magnuson also noted that it had "subordinated its own opinions in a sincere effort to interpret the wishes of the Commission." As a staff we were particularly proud to receive that accolade.

Lowell Reed was most helpful in teaching me how to achieve and express a consensus derived from diverse viewpoints. That entailed listening very carefully to what each person says, noting that person's exact words, and then placing into the consensus document (in our case the Report) precise phrases that the various participants had used in discussion. The technique captures the genuine expressions of the speakers and constitutes a psychological device in that people are inclined to agree with documents that include some of their own words. I learned that taking Reed's advice requires putting one's own sentiments totally aside for the moment in order to completely absorb what the other person is saying. It does not mean totally giving up one's own thoughts, however, because they can be at least partially incorporated into a draft consensus statement that reflects and accurately summarizes what people think and have said.

Russell Lee was always available and advanced many constructive, innovative ideas. He closely associated himself with Lowell Reed in seeking a strong Commission consensus.

Exemplifying the Commission's vision regarding personal health services, the Report recommended that "funds collected through the Old-Age and Survivors Insurance mechanism be utilized to purchase personal health service benefits on a prepayment basis for beneficiaries of that insurance program, under a plan which meets federal standards and which does not involve a means test" (President's Commission, 1952, p. 16). That recommendation materialized only in part some years later as the 1965 Medicare program. The Commission also recommended funds for grants-in-aid to the states to provide personal health services to persons who could not otherwise obtain them—in effect, the subsequent Medicaid program. One cannot, of course, properly infer that such Commission recommendations resulted in the Medicare-Medicaid programs more than a dozen years later, but the Report at least accurately expressed the growing sentiment for their passage.

The Commission issued a very clear statement advocating comprehensiveness of health services to attain health—optimum, physical, mental, and social efficiency and well being—requires more than the cure or alleviation of disease. It requires sound planning in many fields as well as sound health practices and services. Public policies for agriculture, industry, labor, education and welfare, in fact practically all major social and economic plans have implications for health. Although recognizing this fact we have concerned ourselves especially with those measures that are adopted primarily to maintain or improve health. These are: (1) promotion of health, (2) prevention of disease, (3) diagnosis and treatment of disease, (4) rehabilitation. . . . Ideally, they should form a continuum.

The notion of health promotion was expressed as "all of those measures aimed at improving the health aspects of the environment in which people live and at improving personal health practices. . . . Better housing, better nutrition, better working conditions, better education will enhance the health of our people just as certainly as will better physicians' care."

The Commission strongly espoused a larger view of public health, including environmental health and health education as well as personal health services, although it concentrated on the latter. The Report included chapters on professional personal health service personnel, health facilities, organization of personal health services, medical research, and financing personal health services.

Other Experiences in Personal Health Services

After serving as the study director for the President's Commission on Health Needs of the Nation and returning to California, I encountered other opportunities for work in the personal health services field. Governor Brown, in 1959, revived the theme that Earl Warren, as Governor in 1947, had initiated by appointing a Committee on Medical Aid and Health to study the matter. Brown and Warren, the former a Democrat and the latter a Republican, had worked effectively together on many public enterprises during the time that Warren was Governor and Brown was California's Attorney General. Both men held progressive views regarding health. Brown realized that implementing a comprehensive state health plan was not then feasible, as Earl Warren had discovered earlier, so he charged the Committee to (1) study broadly the health needs of citizens, (2) investigate the present provision for, and the cost of, health services, (3) outline a long-range health program and its support, and (4) recommend immediate and specific action to ensure a high standard of health care for all Californians. As chair he appointed the colorful Dr. Roger Egeberg, who was then Medical Director of the Los Angeles County Department of Charities. In its report, presented in December

1960, the Committee recommended regionalizing health services, with councils to plan and coordinate local services; expanding the production of health personnel, especially physicians; increasing the powers of the Boards of Medical and Osteopathic Examiners to establish higher standards of practice; expanding prepayment health service plans; state funding and decentralizing to local governments the operation of major health programs; and state-wide planning of hospital and related facilities and services. The Committee predicted a crisis of unmet needs, lowered quality of care, and inflated costs unless the cooperation of relevant agencies could be obtained for intelligent planning. Although some of the Committee's recommendations were carried out, particularly expanding medical schools and prepayment plans, the failure to plan for and systematically provide the services themselves typified efforts over the past several decades, and the predicted crisis is extending into the twenty-first century (Governor's Committee on Medical Aid and Health, 1960). The California project however, differed from Truman's Health Commission work in two important respects: (1) Egeberg proved to be a much more aggressive leader than Magnuson, and (2) the California Committee emphasized regionalization of health services as a step toward system efficiency.

Another opportunity to become involved in medical care came my way when Governor Brown appointed me to the Public Employees Retirement System (PERS) Board of Administration at the start of the PERS medical program. This program was linked in 1961 to the State's retirement system, but with benefits for active state employees as well as retirees; subsequently, local public employees in California became eligible. I was appointed as one of three new PERS Board members who were specifically designated to develop and oversee regulations for the health program. The legislation provided that employees could choose either a nonprofit health system (Blue Cross/Blue Shield, at that time), a proprietary health insurance policy, or an approved prepaid, capitated medical service plan. This last was then becoming known as a health maintenance organization (HMO). Decades-long favorable experience with the Kaiser-Permanente medical plan by many Californians, and previous experience with the somewhat similar Southern California Ross-Loos plan, made such prepaid capitated medical service organizations especially attractive.

A principal task facing the three new Board members (of whom as the only physician I was the most acquainted with health services) was to assure quality medical service in any HMO that State employees might select. During 1961–1968 the Board tended to approve only well-qualified HMOs for State employees and retirees; in fact, for some years its actions in that regard influenced HMO development in California. During the

Reagan administration and subsequent years, unfortunately, emphasizing their dollar-saving aspects and the failure to preserve a health aim helped stimulate the proliferation of poor-quality HMOs in the state. Though often seemingly inexpensive, they were not providing good quality medical service and apparently had entered the game only for the profits. They and many of their successors have severely tainted the original idea of health maintenance programs. These were often consolidated into huge proprietary enterprises that prioritized financial return to investors rather than their health potential.

My involvement in medical care issues and studies also led to considerable editorial work, including several papers and book chapters, particularly during the 1960s and early 1970s. For the tenth edition of the Rosenau text, editor Philip Sartwell included personal health care as one of the textbook's twelve sections, reflecting a growing acceptance that public health must give the topic systematic attention (Sartwell, 1973). Sartwell also accepted my using "personal health care" rather than "medical care," the term commonly used at the time and still prevailing. The chapter provided an opportunity for me to advance the idea that, in addition to widespread recognition that personal health service can help safeguard health, two other avenues for advancing a population's health must also be followed: environmental measures and influencing behavior.

Environmental and Occupational Health

Most environmental health hazards now arise because we despoil what nature provides, for example, by discharging human sewage into rivers, contaminating natural food while processing and preserving it, and polluting the air with gaseous and particulate wastes. By mid-twentieth century public health environmental concerns were expanding considerably from what they had been decades earlier, when attention was focused almost exclusively on means of controlling the communicable diseases by minimizing sewage pollution of water supplies and requiring appropriate treatment of water for human consumption; seeking pasteurization of milk; and safeguarding food against contamination. Now, rather than focusing almost exclusively on the biological pathogens that are largely coming under control, the technological advances in mining, factory production, transportation, war, and other aspects of life have been creating physical and chemical hazards to health that also require attention. Removing and using materials such as asbestos from the earth, certain chemical manufacturing processes, and other industrial activities have been endangering the health and lives not only of workers but also of those using the products. The 1948 Donora, Pennsylvania, air pollution episode, which caused 20 deaths and made scores of people ill, had demonstrated the danger of airborne chemical and physical agents. The 1952 London episode reinforced that concern; smog in Los Angeles was causing increasing distress and becoming a popular issue (Davis, 2002). Knowledge of occupational exposure to chemicals with adverse health effects was growing, and long-term damage from radiation was appearing among atomic bomb survivors in Japan.

My own interest and activity in environmental aspects of health emerged principally while studying occupational factors in chronic disease. For example, while pursuing possible occupational factors in the lung cancer epidemic in a case–control investigation we identified painters, cooks, and asbestos workers as having an apparently excessive risk of the disease (Breslow, 1955a). Chronic disease epidemiologists commonly undertook such studies in the late 1940s and 1950s. Subsequently tobacco took much higher priority among us, and unfortunately we did not follow up our own findings on occupational factors in lung cancer. Those factors and perhaps other environmental agents may become relatively more prominent in the disease's etiology as the cigarette aspect of the problem diminishes.

Our Bureau of Chronic Disease staff also explored occupational factors in coronary heart disease, which was then commonly attributed to stress of various kinds (Buell & Breslow, 1960). That was the environmental flip side of the psychological type A personality hypothesis that Friedman and Rosenman had advanced. So great was the tendency to accept occupational stress as a principal factor in coronary heart disease that California law early provided workmen's compensation automatically to firemen who suffered from that condition on the grounds that fire fighting itself constituted an occupational hazard for coronary heart disease.

Among other specific groups we studied longshoremen for occupational factors in chronic disease. That investigation surprisingly disclosed that obesity, even more than 40 percent above the Metropolitan Life Insurance Company standard, was not associated with increased risk of heart disease among longshoremen (Buechley, Drake, & Breslow, 1958). The fact that obesity was then regarded as the most preventable factor in heart disease made that anomaly particularly striking, and we wondered why extremely obese longshoremen were spared the hazard of heart disease. Perhaps their work, which previously demanded severe physical exertion but was largely mechanized by the 1950s and thus later required much less physical exertion, coupled with habitual heavy food consumption, had caused long term obesity that did not yield the usual heart disease risk. Subsequently, Ralph Paffenbarger of Stanford used our longshore data to find that physical exertion had protected the men against cardiovascular disease (Paffenbarger, Laughlin, Gima, & Black, 1970). Many investigations have strongly confirmed that physical activity in fact does substantially minimize cardiovascular disease risk.

Air Pollution Control

California experience with environmental health as a big political issue first occurred during the 1954 gubernatorial campaign. Goodwin Knight had succeeded Warren as Governor when the latter was appointed to the U.S. Supreme Court, and was running for a full term against a fairly strong Democratic challenger. The incumbent Knight had to deal with a severe Los Angeles smog episode starting in September 1954, and continuing week after week through October. As the election approached, the smog aroused concern over whether Los Angeles might suffer air pollution fatalities such as had previously occurred in Donora and London. Although coal burning in these other situations obviously generated a different type of air pollution than the Los Angeles smog in which coal burning was minimal, Governor Knight felt compelled to respond to the considerable media attention. After some rather ineffective starts, such as calling on the oil refineries to shut down temporarily, he called upon the State Department of Public Health to answer the question "When does smog become a killer?"

The Bureau of Chronic Disease carried major responsibility for the departmental report which we actually did present to Governor Knight on March 1, 1955 (Bureau of Chronic Disease, 1955). As I noted in a paper published following the investigation of the 1954 episode, "Ordinarily the epidemiologist is confronted with a disease and is asked to determine its source or cause. In the case of smog, he is given an environmental condition and asked to determine whether this causes disease" (Breslow, 1955b, p. 1140). The latter has become a common pattern for epidemiological studies in the environmental health field. Examining available data on both mortality and morbidity yielded no evidence that the 1954 Los Angeles air pollution episode had had any measurable effect on disease occurrence but did reveal a strong, widespread, popular, and professional belief that smog carried an adverse health impact. That notion paralleled the eye and nasal symptoms that many people suffered during smog episodes but that were not included in our assessment of the "killer effects of smog." Our report did emphasize that, although our 1954 health studies had not revealed any immediate smog influence on disease occurrence, even among infants and frail, elderly individuals, the possibility of long-term chronic effects had yet to be studied.

During the 1950s A. J. Haagen-Smit at the California Institute of Technology, while investigating the chemical nature of Los Angeles-type air pollution, demonstrated that the chemical interaction between automobile exhaust and atmospheric ozone in the presence of sunlight constituted its major origin (Haagen-Smit, 1963). The chemical irritant that affected residents accumulated especially under certain weather conditions that favored the chemical reaction and also minimized dispersion of its product by an atmospheric blanket that confined smog close to the ground.

These scientific developments regarding Los Angeles-type air pollution did not receive much further media attention during the 1950s. Popular concern, however, continued. When Pat Brown became Governor in January, 1959, he responded to the fact that smog had again become a considerable public issue, by asking two close aides to assign the problem to the State Department of Public Health. They came directly to John Maga, a Division of Environmental Health engineer, and to me. Maga and I were surprised that top people from the new State administration singled us out personally for the visit, but the assignment they brought really astonished us. Matter of factly and within about a half hour the two Governor's aides charged us with producing a report on California air pollution that would specify (1) ambient (outdoor) air chemical standards that would protect Californians' health, and (2) automobile exhaust standards that would permit achieving these ambient air standards. They brooked no discussion about whether the task would be feasible, whether it could be accomplished within the one year they allowed, or what difficulties might be encountered. The assignment was straightforward. After they left, Maga and I just stared at each other, not quite believing what we had just heard because such a mission then seemed utterly impossible.

With no apparent alternative we adopted the thought that Russell Lee years ago had instilled in my mind: "Just solve the 'impossible' problems." John Goldsmith, an environmental epidemiologist then with the California Department of Public Health, and I collaborated on the task's medical aspects while Maga took over the engineering side. We depended considerably upon expert consultants such as Haagen-Smit because relatively little information that could help us had yet been published. Proceeding systematically to assemble available relevant scientific data, both medical and chemical, we made the necessary estimates and projections and wrote the required report specifying standards for the ambient air and for automobile exhaust. In the course of our work we found it necessary to make some interesting calculations that involved ethical issues. For example, faced with deciding whether to keep carbon monoxide in the ambient air down to a level that would protect cigarette smokers who already were exposed to a considerable self-imposed carbon monoxide risk, we included a carbon monoxide ambient air standard low enough to protect smokers to the extent possible by air pollution control. Equally sensitive calculations were directed toward controlling the several toxic chemicals that automobile exhaust contained.

The State Board of Health meeting in 1960 at which we presented our proposed standards attracted several, probably very high-priced, technical and legal consultants to the automobile and oil industries. The work we reported and the proposed standards, however, drew no criticism. No one spoke a word against the recommendations. Their presence clearly indicated the enormous implications for the automobile and oil industries; however, they acceded to our findings and recommended standards. Moreover they could not challenge the integrity of the State Board of Health which, then chaired by Roger Egeberg, proceeded to adopt the standards. These standards have since been considerably refined to become regulations that the various California air pollution control boards have subsequently implemented. The national Environmental Protection Agency has essentially followed the pattern for air pollution control set by that California project.

Other Experiences in Environmental Health

The United States and Japanese governments established the Atomic Bomb Commission as a joint effort to examine the long-term radiation effects that the atom-bomb blast survivors suffered. The Commission had assembled an excellent staff, and I was privileged to serve on its Medical Advisory Committee. Physical estimates indicated that exposure to the bomb's radiation had decreased in peripheral concentric circles around the blast center, and we found that the harmful health effects, such as the subsequent onset of leukemia, decreased correspondingly among those exposed. The further a person had been situated from the atom bomb's epicenter the less likely was he or she to have suffered health damage. However, no absolute threshold for the radiation's effect on health could be discerned; the diminished effects simply dwindled away. That finding led to the conclusion that, for example, even the tiny radiation exposure that some people receive from natural soil conditions around their homes produces some hazard.

The "no threshold" idea was later extended beyond radiation exposure and became attached to other hazardous physical-chemical environmental conditions. Stimulated by the work of Bruce Ames and other students of the issue, we now realize that this notion appears to have been carried too far. Backlash against the "no threshold" idea applied to environmental hazards other than radiation has unfortunately taken the form of basing environmental control measures largely on the dollar expenditures involved in achieving certain negotiated physical-chemical levels rather than on ascertaining the genuine health effects, how such effects can be controlled, and then achieving the necessary control for human safety. Obviously we must seek some rational approach to the health vs. economics tangle that maintaining healthful environmental conditions now entails, but it appears that the untangling will require some years.

Once having engaged in some environmental health work I have continued participation in that aspect of the field. For example, in the 1970s when I was serving as Dean of the UCLA School of Public Health, a University of California at San Francisco professor of toxicology attracted some highly negative attention from California State legislators because, in effect, he buried one of his findings that was detrimental to some industrial interest and thus neglected the public interest. With University backing I took an appeal to key legislators urging them not to attack the University about the episode but to do something constructive. Coupled with what others did in the same endeavor, that effort proved successful in persuading the Legislature to establish two occupational health centers, one on a northern University of California campus and one in the south, with a million dollars appropriated for each center. At the outset the Legislature gave the responsibility for administering the funds to the State Department of Industrial Relations, not fully trusting the University to maintain the public interest in the occupational-environmental health field. Eventually, full responsibility did devolve upon the University, and by that time we had converted essentially all the available UCLA funds into regular faculty positions. That approach resulted in a strong environmental-occupational health program at UCLA.

During the early 1980s the National Research Council (NRC) established the Committee on Non-Occupational Health Risks of Asbestiform Fibers and asked me to chair it. By that time asbestos had been clearly established as a major occupational hazard. Although the substance had been used since ancient times for various purposes, in the twentieth century huge amounts had been used for insulating buildings, a practice that entailed great exposure of workers who mined and used the asbestos. While that matter was being addressed, physically similar "asbestiform" fibers also came under suspicion. The U.S. Environmental Protection Agency (EPA) sought to reach "a better understanding of the relationship between characteristics of asbestiform fibers and possible adverse health effects from non-occupational exposures," and to that end asked the

NRC to undertake a study. As the NRC Committee, which I chaired, stated in its report, "Large excesses of lung cancer, mesothelioma, pulmonary fibrosis and other pleural abnormalities have been found among workers occupationally exposed to asbestos. Presumably, non-occupational exposures would result in qualitatively similar effects" (Committee on Non-Occupational Health Risks of Asbestiform Fibers, 1984, p. 2). The term "asbestiform fibers" was used in the NRC report "to include both naturally occurring and certain synthetic inorganic and carbon fibers that share some specific physical properties with asbestos" (p. 7). The Committee noted that

> three steps are necessary before one can assess health risk from environmental exposures: determination that a material is toxic and identification of adverse effects; determination of dose–response relationships; and determination of the extent of exposure. At least some types of asbestiform fibers are toxic and have identifiable adverse health effects. However, few occupational studies have demonstrated dose–response relationships, and there is great variability among those few studies. Estimates of exposure outside the workplace are particularly difficult to obtain, and it is the risk from such exposure that is the focus of this report. [pp. 13–14]

The Committee, nevertheless, did make rather crude quantitative risk assessments for non-occupational exposures, using a linear model for low-dose extrapolation (apparently influenced by the "no threshold thesis"), and also qualitative risk assessments for a variety of asbestiform fibers.

My environmental health interests continued into my service on the Los Angeles County Public Health Commission during the late 1990s and beyond. On that Commission we have, among other activities, responsibility for reviewing restaurant inspection and enforcement of sanitation standards in food service. We are also concerned with minimizing children's exposure to lead and other environmental health hazards.

As measures necessary for protection against such dangers have become more complex and large-scale, the federal, state, and local governing bodies have tended to establish responsibility for environmental health services in agencies other than traditional health departments. Thus water safety and sewage disposal typically come under the jurisdiction of local public utilities; air pollution control usually lies in the hands of state and regional air pollution control boards; and protection against occupational health dangers has been assigned to the Occupational Health and Safety Administration (OSHA) of the U.S. Department of Labor and to corresponding State agencies. Another element in the current situation is the fact that, unlike in earlier times when human and animal contamination constituted the major environmental health hazards, most environmental pollution now comes from industrial operations and their products. Regulations to control such pollution often face strong opposition from commercial interests unwilling to make expenditures deemed necessary for the public's health protection. Political tension between environmental health advocates and various commercial interests have thus mounted.

Exclusion of state and local health departments from regulating the environmental health arena has generally favored emphasis on the dollar aspects of each situation rather than its health aspects. Policies tend to reflect mainly how much an offending industry can "afford" rather than how much health protection is involved. Public health should strive to redress the balance now, having failed to maintain the pace of environmental health leadership it established in the early microbiologic era.

The major advantage of environmental health control measures is that, once in place, they do not require any further action on the part of the people being protected. If the food is wholesome, the water properly treated against pathogens and containing adequate fluoride, the air free of pollutants, workplaces safeguarded, housing protected against vermin and injuries, and other aspects of the environment given appropriate attention, health will be protected. Without becoming personally involved people will be secured against many hazards to which they might otherwise be exposed. Of the three ways to protect and maintain health—medical, environmental, and behavioral—only environmental measures entail little or no personal action. In that sense they are still the most effective health measures and have historically yielded the greatest impact.

Influencing Behavior

As the third facet of public health action, health education has long been recognized as essential. It originally consisted largely of trying to persuade individuals to achieve healthful behavior with such slogans as "Don't spit," "See your doctor early in pregnancy," and "Get your children immunized." These were key messages in the campaigns to protect maternity and child health and to combat communicable disease.

By the early 1950s, however, when it became evident that another set of health problems—the chronic diseases—was upon us, public health began to emphasize what was known about the various aspects of people's behavior that were inducing the new epidemics. Obesity had long been identified as a highly significant factor in heart disease, tobacco smoking was being recognized as the major cause of lung cancer, and alcoholism remained a substantial source of liver cirrhosis. What some people did in their everyday lives, such as eating too much, smoking cigarettes, and/ or drinking excessively was contributing to the health situation, just as the ways people had behaved previously (in different situations) had led to earlier health problems. Education in public health, therefore, moved toward controlling the behaviors that investigators were then recognizing as adversely affecting health.

Armed mainly with concepts derived from individual psychology, health educators took up the cudgels against habits that were increasingly determined to be responsible for the noncommunicable diseases. To health educators that still meant persuading people to live in ways that would not endanger health. "Don't smoke" succeeded "Don't spit." Although some efforts had been undertaken decades earlier to combat smoking and excessive drinking, they had been heavily colored with a moralistic approach. Now scientific evidence concerning their role in health damage was providing a different rationale for such endeavors. The main thrust by health educators, however, was still to educate the individuals at risk in the traditional way.

From the beginning of my public health work, going back to training at the University of Minnesota in 1940–1941, health education had appealed to me as a crucial aspect of public health. Leaders in the field at that time certainly extolled it. My own early scientific interest, however, was directed toward discovering what really influenced health-related behavior. My first published study aimed at determining "whether or not the individual who has been immunized against diphtheria or smallpox is more likely to provide for the immunization of his children than is one not so protected, and whether or not the parent who has learned to provide for one child will similarly safeguard other members of the family" (Breslow, Shalit, & Anderson, 1943, p. 384). As reported with caveats, the data indicated that the answer to the first question was negative and to the second, positive.

Experience as the southeastern Minnesota District Health Officer confirmed my belief that what people understood about health underpinned what public health as a social endeavor could accomplish, because what members of a community believed about health seemed far more influential than our technical efforts. Health education as then practiced seemed to build largely on common sense rather than on scientific understanding of what could and should be done about changing health behavior. Seeking to persuade people to adopt healthful behavior consisted largely of conveying information and exhortation. That was the pattern most of us then accepted and followed.

To the extent that health education worked from a scientific base it thus seemed mainly to apply individual psychology in its efforts aimed at encouraging individuals toward healthy personal action, for example, to maintain moderate weight and get health checkups. In 1947, consistent with that approach, I wrote that the health educator "should be called upon to inculcate in the adult and older person the knowledge and motivation which will assist him in prolonging health and avoiding some of the mental and physical infirmity of later years" (Breslow, 1947, p. 280).

Being involved with chronic disease control work in the late 1940s I quickly adopted and helped spread the American Cancer Society's slogans that sought to motivate people's responses to "cancer danger signals" such as a sore that did not heal or tarry stools and to "fight cancer with regular checkups." In the case of heart disease, the public health approach emphasized avoiding obesity and obtaining blood pressure examinations. The voluntary health associations, which were influenced largely by progressive-minded physicians concerned with particular chronic diseases, focused on physician education, public education, and getting people into doctors' offices where preventive services could be initiated, symptoms diagnosed early, and necessary treatment started. Like others in support of voluntary health association work, I joined in encouraging physicians at their conferences and in their journals to educate their patients about actions that would minimize the risk of chronic disease because what people did for themselves seemed as important to their health as what physicians could do for them. I spoke at public meetings that the voluntary health associations organized and meetings of other groups such as unions and churches—wherever one could get onto any group's agenda with health education's chronic disease control message. The impact of such efforts on physicians' and people's conduct, however, did not appear to be great. Although many of us devoted great energy to these activities, we did not seem to be making much headway in persuading individuals to adopt healthful habits, beyond the mostly affluent enthusiasts whom the voluntary health associations reached.

Personal Responsibility vis-a-vis Conditions of Life

The extent to which we then passively accepted the conditions of life that were profoundly influencing behavior rather than analyzing and dealing with them may be seen in the following:

Self-control was a popular idea a few decades ago; it is somewhat neglected now, but will be required more than ever in what has come to be called the affluent society. Perhaps, the term self-control is out of fashion and will never be popular again. The practice of something like it, however, is essential to good health when food, liquor, cigarettes, and automobiles are so widely available and physical demand on their users minimal.

How man uses these good things of life determines health far more completely than all the work physicians do. Helping people live in this situation is a major task of health education in this era. . . . [Breslow, 1968, p. 794]

Like others at the time I emphasized helping people live in their situations and resist any adverse impact on behavior rather than trying to change the situations that we now realize were producing such harmful health behavior and its consequences.

As this trend gained momentum, opposition mounted against what was called "blaming the victims." Why focus on "the poor devils," it was argued, when they really can't help themselves? Some of the previous moralistic tone as well as the backlash against it continued. As knowledge began to accumulate concerning the role of health habits in the modern health scene, emphasis on health-related behavior intensified and the focus on individuals prevailed despite objections to blaming the victim. On that issue, the President's Commission on Health Needs of the Nation stated,

The individual effort of an informed person will do more for his health and that of his family than all of the things that can be done for them. In the past, measures for health maintenance demanded individual responsibility only to a limited degree. The development of pure water supplies, pasteurization of milk and other sanitary accomplishments were achieved through social action in which the individual may have participated as a citizen, but was required to take no further individual responsibility.

Future accomplishments, however, depend to an even greater degree upon the individual's assumption of responsibility for his own health. It is the individual who must consult his physician for early care, avoid obesity and alcoholism, and drive his automobile safely. These things cannot be done for him. They require both information and motivation.

Recognition of the significance of the individual responsibility for health does not discharge the obligation of a society that is interested in the health of its citizenry. Such recognition, in fact, increases social responsibility for health. Heretofore, social effort on behalf of health has been limited largely to such measures as delivery of pure water to the individual's tap and the sanitary disposal of his sewage. Now it becomes necessary for a society which wishes to advance the health of its citizens to adopt measures that will guarantee to the individual an opportunity to make appropriate decisions on behalf of his health. Society must assure its citizens access to professional services, education concerning personal health practices, and a reasonably safe physical environment. Only then can individual responsibility for health exercised through personal action reach its full potential.[President's Commission on Health Needs of the Nation, 1952, p. 8]

Those last three sentences constitute an important element of current public health philosophy. Biologically we possess an instinct to protect our individual lives and health. Still, as social beings interested in community health protection, it is also essential that we assure opportunity for and encourage individual decisions that are conducive to health, provide a healthful physical environment, and make available high quality personal health services.

As we realized more and more fully that the twentieth-century epidemics of chronic disease, with their extensive damage to health, resulted from certain habit patterns, we began to seek more effective ways of dealing with the problem. We gradually began to see that influencing individual choices in these matters was not the only or even the most fruitful approach to the situation. The habit patterns were merely responses to certain conditions of life, and we realized that we should be directing attention to those conditions themselves. Production and marketing of cigarettes was the outstanding example. Manufacturing and distributing that form of tobacco was essentially a twentieth-century phenomenon and was producing the well-known health hazard. The highly sophisticated marketing that incorporated what the tobacco companies (then secretly) knew about its addictive properties was the major condition that had to be attacked (Glantz, Slade, Bero, Hanauer, & Barnes, 1996).

Rather than focusing effort on individual responses to the conditions in which people live it is probably more effective to deal with the conditions themselves. Exemplifying the impact of that mode of action, voluntary health agency use of television proved so effective in retarding cigarette use that the tobacco companies gave up their television advertising in trade for no further voluntary health agency attacks on the industry by television. Further illustrating this strategy, the California tobacco control program in the 1990s successfully directed considerable effort to television messages that discourage smoking. That program has also accomplished the prohibition of smoking in public buildings, restaurants, and bars; and restricting access to tobacco products in vending machines and retail stores that make cigarettes available to young people. The focus is thus on the conditions that favor smoking rather than on the smokers themselves. (This issue will be addressed further in chapter 7 on Tobacco Control.)

In the case of other health-related habits, public health encounters multiple forces rather than a single industry and its allies. For example, influences on physical exertion include reduction of physical demands at work and the opportunities for exercise breaks on the job. Similar opportunities at school and availability of places to exercise in neighborhoods are also important. Dealing with health-related habits is thus evolving into a socioecological strategy for advancing health that departs sharply from the older view that individual behaviors adverse to health should be combated mainly by approaching the individuals. Avoiding harmful habits and adopting healthful ones has always been a health aim, but concentrating on individuals really did mean in effect blaming the victims. That narrow perspective on lifestyle as a factor in disease causation failed to consider that behavior consists of patterns in the circumstances of one's life. They are not simply a matter of personal volition in a vacuum.

The commonly expressed argument that people have an individual right to engage in behavior that may injure their health depends on the notion that the behavior does not injure others. That notion is already crumbling in the case of excessive alcohol consumption where evidence is accumulating concerning the direct adverse impact on others. Though less direct, such impact is also appearing in the case of obesity, for example, in narrow airplane seats and in the socially shared costs of medical care whereby people pay for medical services for others as well as themselves; for example, people of moderate weight help pay for the excessive costs of those who are overweight.

Fundamental biological factors, of course, also enter into the health-related habit situation. For people who have long been deprived of certain "good things" and then rather suddenly are able to obtain them, fatty and sweet foods are tasty; nicotine and other drugs create physiological satisfactions; and people quickly grasp opportunities to rest, thus minimizing physical exertion. By tolerating marketing that encourages people to indulge these biological propensities we have socially neglected the circumstances that result in behavior that is adverse to health.

A SOCIAL ECOLOGY FOR HEALTH

To counter the decades-long tendency to ignore the circumstances that influence behavior it is becoming necessary to alter people's life situations by constraining the marketing of nicotine and other drugs, promoting the use of healthful foods instead of those that are unhealthy, and making space and opportunity available to all for physical exercise. Such a social ecology strategy would change from health-negative to health-positive those aspects of the social and physical environments that influence health-related behavior, including the visual and auditory messages that now reach people. The social milieu would thus emphasize pro-health rather than anti-health influences. Instead of allowing nutrition lessons in the classroom to be eroded by the realities in the lunchroom, an appropriate strategy is to influence the actual conditions in the school lunchroom—the vending machines, the cafeteria menu, and the food marketing—toward healthfulness. California, for example, has recently enacted legislation to remove sweet sodas from the school lunchroom, and some school districts are already replacing vending machine sodas with milk and fruit juices.

The current anti-tobacco movement, particularly in California and a few other states, has already adopted this social ecology strategy. My participation in that program has provided insight into the intricacies of such effort. The adversely affected industry fights viciously against actions that oppose marketing of its product, even though that product clearly contributes extensively to morbidity and mortality. The counter-attack by the industry employs potent weaponry such as large-scale funding of legislators' election campaigns and other means of seeking legislative action favorable to the industry. The moderate successes against tobacco have stimulated efforts against guns in which a similar battle is shaping up against the industry factor in violence, and a comparable solution is appearing in aspects of the nutrition situation. Fortunately, some elements of the food industry seem to have learned from other industry marketing experiences and are already joining the social health movement to the extent of at least adding healthful menu items to their traditional unhealthful ones.

A social ecology strategy thus complements the long-standing physical ecology for public health. The latter embraces such items as fluoridating water to save teeth and adding iodine to salt to minimize thyroid disease, actions directed toward improving conditions that affect bodily tissues. Social ecology for health consists of establishing conditions that favor healthful personal behavior. It can produce a milieu in which people are encouraged rather than discouraged (as often is the case now) to act in ways that enhance health.

Fulfilling the public health mission, assuring "conditions in which people can be healthy" (in the words of the Institute of Medicine) thus requires attention to all three conditions: (1) the availability of personal health services (i.e., medical and related care), (2) environmental health (i.e., physical ecology), and (3) behavioral influences (i.e., mainly social ecology). Experience gained in public health, especially during the latter half of the twentieth century, has yielded this concept of how to advance the public's health. People engaged in the field may be personally involved in only one or another of its three aspects. Their work, however, can be enhanced by understanding how the other arms of public health contribute to their aim and collaborating with them. Those aspiring to leadership in the field would do well to understand and vigorously espouse all three aspects of public health. As fundamentally a social enterprise, public health entails politics and not infrequently political struggles in order to achieve the "condition in which people can be healthy."

Concepts, Determinants, and Measurement of Health and Role of the Human Population Laboratory

6

INTRODUCTION

Primitive man attributed diseases and trauma, as he did unwanted things generally, to demons and evil spirits. Whether battle injury or some illness occurred, the ancients regarded such events as expressions of some nonmaterial force. Health adversities were thus thought to reflect encounters with "bad" spirits. Some religious people still appeal for disease prevention or recovery to "good" but nonmaterial forces.

Currently dominant Western thought on these matters, however, is said to have originated about 400 B.C. on the Greek island of Cos where Hippocrates and other physicians began to regard disease as a process of nature, not the result of evil spirits (Sigerist, 1943).

Hippocrates and Other Early Thinkers

Hippocrates, who is often acclaimed as "the father of medicine," considered health to be a set of bodily conditions that one's behavior and the environment strongly influenced. That still persists as our principal Western concept thought about health. We have advanced considerably in detailing the three elements and their relationships—the body and its function, environment, and behavior—but the basic scheme remains the same. Hippocrates advanced the view that climate and other environmental factors substantially affected one's health. Harmony between a

95

person and his environment was the ideal that healthful eating, drinking, sexual practices, work, and recreation could help achieve. Early Chinese thought emphasized similar notions. Ancient physicians also believed that balance among four bodily humors—blood, phlegm, yellow bile, and black bile—represented health in the biologic sense. (Now, we often measure blood sugar, cholesterol, and the like as one way to ascertain the degree of health.)

The Cartesian Paradigm

During the Middle Ages the Cartesian paradigm emerged, that is, the view that human creatures as well as other things in the universe function as machines. Hence, helping people maintain health required that one must study anatomy and physiology to determine how the body functions, understand what particular agents and mechanisms cause dysfunction, and then subdue those agents or their effects in order to prevent or treat the diseases that result therefrom. That mechanistic concept has nurtured modern medicine's development, which has evolved principally by using the Cartesian notion in responding to each era's health problems.

As noted in chapter 4, communicable diseases were the overwhelming public health burden during the early industrial era. Epidemics of plague, smallpox, and other diseases had swept over various and sometimes large populations in the preceding centuries. They continued to do so while tuberculosis, pneumonia, and dysentery became endemic in the factory towns to which people flocked from the countryside for jobs and other nineteenth- and early twentieth-century opportunities. Social observers in the mid-nineteenth century regarded the crowding, filth, exhausting work, and poor nutrition as key factors in the high mortality among the new urban residents. Reformers with an ecological view sought to improve those conditions as a way to advance health and life generally, even though not much had yet been learned about the precise origins and mechanisms of disease. Death certificates listed the major communicable diseases of early industrial society as the leading causes of death into the twentieth century because reforms came so slowly.

Substantial progress against disease was achieved based on the Cartesian model. As early as 1796 the English country physician, Edward Jenner, noticed that dairy maids had smooth skin and reasoned that their good fortune in not being pockmarked by smallpox might result from having been exposed to cowpox, a common disease of cattle, by contact while milking. When transmitted to humans, it creates only a single pustule at the point of infection and only rarely any significant

adverse consequences, but it stimulates immunity to the biologically related human disease, smallpox. The dairy maids did not become pockmarked from the multiple pustules of smallpox because early encounters
with cowpox made them immune to the more serious infection. This
observation not only led Jenner to develop vaccination against smallpox
with cowpox vaccine, but it also advanced a new idea: creating immunity
to particular diseases. Implementing that idea has yielded, among other
benefits, the world-wide eradication of smallpox, which has been our
first success in literally wiping out a disease. The idea of vaccine-induced
immunity has further resulted in vastly reducing other communicable
diseases such as diphtheria and pertussis, and the prospect of eradicating
others such as poliomyelitis and measles.

Pursuing the mechanistic strategy also generated the germ theory of
disease and the spectacular successes based on it. Technological advances
such as the microscope permitted identifying bacteria and other disease
organisms; further, they allowed Robert Koch and others to establish the
science of bacteriology. Scientists following its precepts, and modifying
and extending them, have thus ascertained what distinct microbic or
submicrobic agents—viruses and parasites (and now prions) as well as
bacteria—are responsible for certain diseases. They also discovered how
these agents spread through the environment and infect humans. For
example, the old notion that miasms from swampy land ("bad air")
caused malaria has been replaced by our understanding that plasmodia
carried by mosquitoes (which grow in the swamps) infect people and
thus constitute the environment-generated disease mechanism. Finding
such disease mechanisms—the external agents, their transmission to
humans, and their pathogenic paths in the body—has inspired medical
scientists during recent decades to tackle noncommunicable as well as
communicable diseases in somewhat the same manner, that is, identifying
various disease agents, how they reach humans, and their mechanisms
of action in the body.

Conditions of Life

Concentrating so exclusively on this successful aspect of improving health,
however, has diverted attention from how the larger environment pro-
motes disease and finding how such adverse social conditions as poverty
and poor schooling can be overcome to improve health as well as life
generally. By adopting the Cartesian paradigm as almost the sole approach to disease, the scientific establishment has thus far devoted too
little consideration to the broader physical and social environmental

origins of disease and the means of attacking them. Emphasizing specific disease agents and mechanisms has obviously yielded immense benefits in communicable disease control, but, as Thomas McKeown (1976) has pointed out, the improvement against tuberculosis, for example, has mainly reflected progress against adverse living circumstances such as poor nutrition and crowding. These broader approaches have also achieved noncommunicable disease control, at least as much as pursuing mechanistic pathways has.

Consider tobacco consumption, which has recently been responsible for about one-fifth of all deaths in the United States, mainly through affecting the lung, blood vessels, and heart. Discovering such relationships received a tremendous boost from epidemiological studies proving that smoking causes lung cancer and is a major factor in coronary heart disease. Seeking to know which specific components of tobacco smoke stimulate what bodily changes leading to lung cancer and coronary heart disease has thus far produced relatively little for the struggle against those conditions. In fact, promoting such Cartesian-based efforts has been used to erect obstacles against disease control because they have enabled some policy makers to postpone necessary action by asserting that more research to discover precise mechanisms is needed. Some scientists have supported these decisions, claiming that only knowing a mechanistic cause can justify definitive action.

The lung cancer epidemic has resulted from commercially exploiting a technological innovation (cigarette manufacturing), linking sales of the product to nicotine addiction, and using the media and political processes both to promote and sustain sales and to block counteraction. Combating the epidemic, which is now being undertaken in the United States and some other countries, and stopping its spread in the developing world is a social task that will yield no likely foreseeable benefit from determining which precise physical or chemical agent or agents induce what changes in the pulmonary cells that progress to lung cancer. Certainly it is not sensible to await knowledge of such detailed mechanisms, as some have proposed, before proceeding with control of smoking.

We are thus beginning to realize that major harm to health in the United States and other industrialized countries still arises out of the conditions of life. That is why the Institute of Medicine has defined public health's mission as "fulfilling society's interest in assuring the conditions in which people can be healthy" (Institute of Medicine, 1988, p. 7).

It is clear that the twentieth century's greatest epidemic, coronary heart disease, arose out of the conditions of life. That disease's major fatal manifestation, myocardial infarction, was first recognized in the United States during the early part of the century. The disease reached a peak during the early 1960s when it caused about one-third of all deaths in the United States. Fortunately, it has since been steadily and substantially declining. We now realize that coronary heart disease results from several conditions of life that have characterized the industrial era: increased availability and consumption of animal fat, lessened physical exertion, availability and consumption of cigarettes, and social influences leading to hypertension. Vulnerability to these several factors, of course, varies according to genetic and other influences among individuals, but the disease results when exposure to such conditions induces people to overburden their bodily capacity to withstand the assault on the coronary arteries and avoid the resulting damage. Our bodies simply do not have the resources to cope with overexposing ourselves to the conditions that have affected us so adversely. The epidemic occurs first among the more affluent members of society because they are the first to encounter the adverse conditions; it then descends through the social ranks to reach the less affluent as they gradually become exposed to the same conditions. The more affluent people meanwhile recognize and begin avoiding the causative conditions, and they also benefit the most from significant therapeutic advances.

Coronary heart disease is thus as classic a social disease as tuberculosis, though resulting from quite different underlying conditions of life and having a different social gradient. It starts at the top and descends through the social strata within nations and the socioeconomic ranks among nations. Not only do poorer American men currently suffer the epidemic most severely, but developing nations are now encountering it and the most affluent there become the first affected. The rise and fall of coronary heart disease has thus reflected the social conditions that determine its occurrence, and control is accomplished mainly by ascertaining and dealing with these conditions. Knowledge of the detailed pathologic mechanisms has helped somewhat, especially in treatment, but it plays a considerably lesser role in overall control.

Having achieved substantial though by no means complete control of the communicable diseases and growing control of the noncommunicable diseases, we can now envision a new concept of health. People are living longer. Also, human life, especially in the developed countries, is far less disease burdened than in previous times. Steadily declining age-specific disability rates have occurred during recent decades in the United States.

Well-Being

The World Health Organization (WHO) founders defined health anew, as "physical, mental and social well-being, not merely the absence of disease and infirmity" (World Health Organization, 1948). In previous decades overcoming or preventing pathologic changes had dominated the health field because the health problem facing society, and medicine in particular, had been combating disease. Attaining health certainly includes conquering disease, but the WHO concept acknowledges that as being only part of the goal. A positive aspect of health, "well-being," also comes onto the agenda. This idea reflected the fact that even though many people have suffered chronic illness in recent decades and their numbers have been increasing as the population ages, more people have also been living beyond the once-allotted "three-score and ten" with an increasing proportion of them largely escaping diseases and infirmity. As that group has expanded and younger people likewise experience less disability, it becomes apparent that people's health aim could and should exceed "merely the absence of disease and infirmity."

The three dimensions of well-being, "physical, mental, and social," constituted a second noteworthy aspect of the WHO health definition. Health thinking had long incorporated the first two, although understanding of the mental dimension had not advanced very far. Social well-being was a different notion whose meaning was by no means clear. These separate dimensions of well-being, however, attracted little attention from the scientific community; in fact the WHO concept came to be generally regarded as a slogan, not subject to scientific use. Because the concept seemed so ill-defined, "woolly" as some called it, applying it in health investigations with quantitative methods appeared farfetched.

Another WHO statement, the 1986 Ottawa Charter, asserted health to be "a resource for everyday living." In this view health is neither a balance nor a state, but a "capacity" of one's being. Not just a bodily, mental, or social condition, it includes the competence to cope with the conditions of life and the ability to "realize aspirations and satisfy needs" (World Health Organization-Europe, 1986). The Ottawa Charter thus defines health as even beyond well-being. It also expresses a more measurable condition than the original WHO definition.

This brief account of ideas about health and its determinants has indicated some of its main aspects. It is an extremely complex subject; people's views about it have varied tremendously and no consensus has yet been reached, nor does one seem likely to be reached soon. One can, however, discern a strong trend in recent decades toward including in the concept of health something beyond the absence of disease, and the idea of health determinants is beginning to mean something beyond specific agents of disease and their mechanisms.

MEASUREMENT OF HEALTH

Until fairly recently actual measurement of a population's health consisted almost exclusively of compiling physician reports of births, deaths, and communicable diseases, and relating the numbers thus assembled to census data covering various geographic areas. These statistics permitted keeping track of death and disease rates according to age, gender, and various other categories; how long people lived; and morbidity and mortality from the principal communicable diseases. Incidence, and especially epidemics of the latter were the major, generally accepted public health problems until the mid-twentieth century. As noncommunicable diseases became more prominent, however, it became necessary to consider how they and their impact on society could be measured. Their relationship to conditions of life also became a problem. Such issues were emerging in public health circles at the mid-century point.

As early as 1916–1920 United States Public Health Service epidemiologists had been exploring new approaches to investigating and measuring disease and its correlates in populations. They were trying to get beyond using only data reported by physicians and applying thereto the microbial theory of disease causation. For example, Joseph Goldberger pursued pellagra's origin and its high prevalence in the southeastern states by studying its relationship to the way people lived there and especially what they ate. He adopted an ecologic view for his work rather than simply using the prevailing notion that the disease originated from some infectious agent. This approach led Goldberger to propose a dietary causation and to use an experiment that would prove his hypothesis, namely, that nutritional inadequacy was responsible for the disease. In a children's institution where the disease was endemic he simply supplemented the regular but poor diet for some of the children with milk and other more nourishing food. He then observed that pellagra disappeared among the better nourished children whereas the disease continued among those eating only the regular, institutional diet. Together with Edgar Sydenstriker, Goldberger also surveyed households in southern cotton mill villages to ascertain and demonstrate the broad relationships among disability, nutrition, and economic conditions (Goldberger, 1964).

In the new health situation, individuals often suffered from multiple chronic diseases which sometimes ended in death. For example, diabetes, heart disease, and arthritis could all be responsible for ill health in the same person. It thus seemed important to determine how morbidity in a generic sense, and not only particular diseases, arose in a population. Some of those concerned with health measurement began to measure morbidity as a non–disease-specific phenomenon, aiming to find and use better health indices for delineating the health problems confronting contemporary industrialized society. Just as previous health indices had clarified the communicable disease tasks of earlier days, the emerging problems required health measurement methodology that would permit monitoring progress in controlling morbidity in a generic sense. The new health situation emphasized the disability that resulted from one or more pathologic conditions or specific diseases. Days lost from work and the need for care because of disabling conditions were impeding both industrial productivity and the personal enjoyment of life.

In one significant respect the new efforts to measure health and its determinants paralleled long-established health measurement methods, that is, they related health phenomena to geographically defined populations. Investigators however, often rejected the common notion that the chronic diseases were inherent in the aging process and the inevitable consequence of it. Following the earlier mortality and disease-specific indices, the evolving morbidity studies also concentrated on specific groups within a larger population. This stance guided several sickness surveys in the United States and elsewhere (i.e., obtaining morbidity information reported by a sample of people representing a total population and particular segments of it). Such surveys often sought the resultant social impact such as work disability or days in the hospital and sometimes encompassed disease-specific phenomena as reported by the persons surveyed, for example, heart disease or asthma.

The first substantial measurement of a population's health using such a morbidity survey was undertaken in Hagerstown, Maryland, in 1921–1924 by the U.S. Public Health Service and the Hagerstown Health Department (Sydenstriker and Brundage, 1925). It covered 1,822 white families, a third of the total population, with periodic household informant interviews every 6–8 weeks for 29 months designed to ascertain disabling and nondisabling, acute and chronic illness. The fact that checking local medical records largely corroborated information that individuals reported in the Hagerstown studies indicated that the household survey method could credibly depict a community's sickness profile.

Several such morbidity surveys took place during the period 1928–1943, with the participation of the U.S. Public Health Service: one covering mostly urban localities located in 18 states; and others in Cattaraugus County, New York; the Eastern Health District of Baltimore, Maryland; and elsewhere (Collins, 1951). From these surveys a picture of a population's health status emerged beyond the one that mortality and communicable disease reporting systems revealed. A depression enterprise undertaken by the Works Project Administration constituted the largest such investigation, the 1935–1936 National Health Survey covering 700,000 families. It aimed at job creation as well as health measurement, focusing on disabling conditions that kept people from their usual activities. The household sample survey method using self-reports of sickness and related data proved to be effective for assessing the extent and nature of a population's total morbidity. Of considerable significance, that method embraced noncommunicable conditions and morbidity therefrom and thus facilitated the break from the concept that communicable diseases were the only public health problem.

As these ideas were emerging and being tried during the 1920s and beyond, the strong links among voluntary health agency spokespersons, biomedical scientists, and Congressional leaders was laying the foundation for the vast National Institutes of Health development, starting with the National Cancer Institute, then the National Heart Institute, followed by a succession of others. Funds thus made available nourished and reinforced traditional biomedical and mechanistic approaches to disease control. Medical centers responded to the availability of funds by initiating biological investigations related to specific disease mechanisms, for example, the possible role of viruses in cancer. Meanwhile, the various health organizations devoted to cancer, heart disease, poliomyelitis, and other specific disease problems mobilized public interest and action. Biomedical research efforts thus continued to mount and dovetailed neatly with the popular and legislative concern with particular diseases.

However, other trends in thinking about health persisted. As people aged and the burden of their chronic illnesses increased, the need for long-term care expanded and the total dollar cost of services for the chronically disabled rose dramatically. Because the services were directed mainly toward helping patients deal with their physical and mental impairments, the particular disease pathologies did not matter much. The idea of chronic illness in a generic sense thus escalated along with the medical focus on particular diseases.

At the same time the idea that medicine encompassed more than the application of biomedical science was stirring some circles. Sigerist, the medical historian, commented: "That medicine is a social science sounds like a truism, yet it cannot be repeated often enough because in medical education we still act as if medicine were a natural science and nothing else. There can be no doubt that the target of medicine is to keep individuals adjusted to their environment as useful members of society, or re-adjust them when they have dropped out as a result of illness. It is a social goal . . . " (Sigerist, 1943).

Such thinking suggested that paths to health beyond traditional avenues should be aggressively explored. That did not mean abandoning the scientific method, but rather applying it to aspects of health other than the pathological mechanisms of disease. Before that break from tradition could occur, however, a new concept of health and a method of measuring it were necessary.

START OF MY OWN THINKING

The bold WHO 1948 view intrigued me as a possible opening to a new way of thinking about health. It not only inspired my interest in the definition of health but also raised questions about what should be done about it during the latter half of the twentieth century and perhaps beyond. In particular, I wondered whether one could use the WHO concept for the scientific investigation of health despite the prevailing negative view of that question.

Besides these stirrings about the definition of health, several other trends led me in the California Department of Public Health to develop what became the Human Population Laboratory in Alameda County. For one thing, the idea that current disease problems stemmed largely from people's living conditions was attracting many young physicians, myself included. The long-established link between social disadvantage— poverty, racial and ethnic discrimination, poor education—and health was receiving renewed emphasis. Indigent people not only suffered higher levels of tuberculosis and other communicable diseases, but they were also burdened with more high blood pressure, heart disease, cancer, and higher morbidity and mortality in general. Although the "New Deal" and subsequent high employment during World War II had alleviated the Great Depression's consequences somewhat, the economically and educationally disadvantaged segments of the population continued to experience substantially poorer health than more affluent people. The obvious social origins of poor health did not seem remediable by determining the biologic mechanisms of disease. More direct approaches to the external causes seemed necessary.

Furthermore, identifying cigarette smoking as the principal cause of the lung cancer epidemic and a substantial factor in coronary heart disease supported the idea that social conditions and people's responses to them were responsible for much ill health. The production and marketing of cigarettes exemplified such social conditions, and people's responses were buying and smoking them. The fact that people continued smoking, of course, resulted in part from the biological phenomenon of addiction. Discovery that smoking caused so much disease, together with the earlier finding that obesity hastened mortality, stimulated thinking that poor health generally reflected conditions in which certain ways of living prevailed. That notion differed from the one that medical students learned as Koch's postulates for determining the causes of disease, that is, identifying and confirming a biologic organism as the responsible agent. That previous model now seemed outmoded as the exclusive pattern for ascertaining disease causation because experience with smoking had clearly demonstrated that one could scientifically determine causation without knowing the precise agent or its mode of action and control disease by using that knowledge concerning the origin of disease.

Still another factor favoring new ways of studying health emerged from measurement science. Extending physician reporting to all the human health conditions, in effect a continuing universal health census, was obviously impractical. If the WHO concept were to be adopted as a health goal toward which progress would be measured, perhaps systematic sampling could ascertain a population's health in a generic sense, for which the U.S. Public Health Service disability surveys in the 1930s had pointed the way.

Reliance on sampling methods required assurance that they would produce data accurately, or at least to a specified degree. Fortunately, considerable headway was being made in survey research methodology, especially in tracking public opinion on political and commercial topics. The American Association of Public Opinion Research (AAPOR) brought together the statisticians who were using survey methods. Applying these methods to health measurement, however, raised questions such as whether people could and would report their health conditions as accurately as they might be willing to report less personal information.

Although ultimately aimed at measuring health in the WHO sense, our first efforts toward health measurement in the California Department of Public Health were much more modest. Termed the California Morbidity Research Project, they consisted of surveys designed to measure the population's morbidity and medical care services. We began in 1948 to explore various means of measuring chronic disease morbidity in California as a part of our chronic disease control program (Breslow & Ott, 1954; Breslow & Mooney, 1956). A grant from the National Institutes of Health enabled us in 1950 to test the household sample survey method for that purpose. Whether people could or would report their health conditions was a major issue. A pilot study conducted in San Jose revealed that people did report their health status and services substantially the same as what physician, hospital, and disability insurance records indicated (Breslow, 1954).

Meanwhile, as noted earlier, the Commission on Chronic Illness had undertaken health surveys combined with medical examinations in rural

Hunterdon County, New Jersey and urban Baltimore, Maryland (Commission on Chronic Illness 1957 and 1959). The substantial U.S. Public Health Service sample survey method experience, the Commission on Chronic Illness surveys, and other studies yielded sufficient basis for President Eisenhower in 1956 to approve a United States Public Health Service recommendation to establish the National Health Survey on a regular, periodic basis. It became another major element in monitoring the American people's health.

During 1954–1955, based upon satisfactory pilot health survey experience, we undertook the California Morbidity Survey involving a sample of 12,000 households with 35,000 persons, representing the entire state's population (Breslow, 1957; Breslow & Mooney, 1956). In that project, conducted via a contract with the United States Census Bureau, we utilized statistical expertise from the Census Bureau, which had become heavily involved in population sampling, and from the U.S. Public Health Service. The information collected in that survey yielded several reports concerning health in California; for example, "An Epidemiological Investigation of Coronary Heart Disease" (Drake, Buechley, & Breslow, 1957). A further survey in 1956 provided data for studies related to various California Department of Public Health interests such as air pollution health effects (Breslow & Goldsmith, 1958).

The Public Health Service drew upon its experience with the California Morbidity Survey in launching the National Health Survey in 1957. We joined forces with that Survey in order to obtain information specifically for California. The resulting monograph (California Department of Public Health, 1958) revealed the extent to which various conditions affected people, the disability they caused in several groups as well as in the whole population, and the associated medical and hospital services.

THE HUMAN POPULATION LABORATORY CONCEPT

Considering what health meant, how to measure it, the developing knowledge of how to achieve it, and the methodological advances in the nascent health survey experience led me to envision and establish a Human Population Laboratory for investigating health as the WHO defined it and the ways of living that largely influence it. We located it in Alameda County, California where the State Department of Public Health was then headquartered. The County included approximately one million persons who were fairly similar to the nation's demographic profile, making it a suitable situation for such a project.

Because the term "Human Population Laboratory" sometimes provokes either curiosity or antipathy, explaining the original concept seems desirable. *Webster's Seventh New Collegiate Dictionary* (1963) defines laboratory as "a place providing opportunity for experimentation, observation, or practice in a field of study." A laboratory for health research usually connotes a space where scientists work on various projects using glassware, centrifuges, and other equipment to discover means of preventing or curing disease. Epidemiology using survey data is another type of health research: investigating the natural history of disease by studying it where people actually live. A Human Population Laboratory is a place for measuring health and systematically examining how the ways people live relate to their health. It differs from a biochemistry or virus laboratory in that its research staff investigates the entire population as it lives in a defined geographic area, rather than focusing on some disease mechanism. It also differs in that experiments are not performed; instead, reliance is placed on observing natural phenomena related to health including whatever human behavior seems relevant. It resembles a biochemistry or virus laboratory, however, in its substantial effort toward developing and testing methods for observing and measuring the phenomena being studied and in the research staff's engagement in a variety of projects, organized as a research program. Human Population Laboratory may, of course, be an imperfect term.

Throughout history, disease and premature death have resulted not only from man's poor understanding of his natural environment and how to control it, but also from various conditions he has created in that environment. Ironically, many disease-causing conditions result from man's effort to improve his life. To exchange goods with people living far away and thus develop international commerce, men took long voyages during which they acquired scurvy. To build industrial society people crowded together and thereby accelerated the spread of certain communicable diseases, notably tuberculosis. To establish and implement the Western lifestyle, people have subjected themselves to factors whose consequence is coronary heart disease.

Recent epidemiological work has made clear that not only can one factor be involved in several different pathological conditions, but also one condition can result from any or a combination of several factors. For example, lung cancer develops from certain occupational exposures, such as to asbestos, as well as from cigarette smoking; moreover, asbestos can also cause the disease asbestosis. Pneumonia follows exposure to a variety of organisms and chemicals that also cause diseases other than pneumonia. Congenital malformations appear to have multiple causes. Hence, the notion of a sine qua non for each and every disease must be put aside.

Increasing interest in measuring general morbidity arose mainly from the desire to use it as a basis for delineating socioenvironmental factors responsible for health status. Other investigators studied measures of the effectiveness of medical service, called "outcomes research," to determine what medical services were actually accomplishing. They introduced such terms as "sickness impact profile" to express essentially what others were calling general morbidity. Hans Selye advocated studying the "syndrome of just being sick" (Selye, 1952). It thus seemed desirable to measure population health in a generic sense, consider its demographic correlates, and examine its relationship to particular aspects of living that might be responsible for ill health. It was hoped that such aspects of living would be amenable to change as a means of improving health. Disease specificity had largely sufficed as the basis for health advance as long as one microbe appeared to cause mainly one disease, but disease processes, certainly the noncommunicable conditions and even those linked to specific microbic organisms, were more and more proving to be multifactorial.

Meanwhile, as we in California undertook morbidity studies and methodological investigations to improve their quality, a new idea was emerging. Could we measure health itself and not just its negative, that is, the diseases and morbidity that followed pathology? Could we now go beyond morbidity and approach health quantitatively? As noted earlier, the World Health Organization's health concept, "physical, mental, and social well-being, not merely absence of disease and infirmity," had been generally regarded merely as rhetoric, not subject to scientific use. Using the population sample survey technique, however, opened the possibility of applying the World Health Organization definition to determining the health of populations. Surveys had already begun to yield data about morbidity and its disability consequences without regard to disease classifications. Investigators were finding how much general morbidity occurred in the population as a whole; its distribution according to age, gender, social class, and ethnic segments; and what factors were associated with it and might be causing it. In the course of these studies during the 1950s it occurred to me that we might quantify the opposite—health—as well as morbidity. The challenge really came from the WHO definition. Could we use it scientifically to measure health in the same way as we measured general morbidity?

My basic thought was that we should look upon health status as a spectrum, ranging from very good to very poor. Every living person could be placed somewhere on a health status spectrum, which would extend from disability that severely impaired living at one end, through various points, all the way to great energy for living and thus excellent health at the other. Using such a spectrum, one might measure not only individual health but also a population's health and how people of particular age, gender, and other categories congregate on the spectrum. Older people, for example, would generally fall toward one end and young adults toward the other. Perhaps factors such as obesity, excess alcohol consumption, education, and income level would be measurably associated with health status. Significant factors in health, morbidity, and mortality—all potentially alterable by social means—could thus be identified.

That concept, however, encountered strong resistance. During the 1950s and thereafter the laboratory and clinical biomedical sciences were flourishing in America, spurred by increasing Congressional appropriations to the National Institutes of Health, which then passed a large portion of the funds for health research on to universities and institutes around the country. Prospects for discovering more and more vaccines and penicillin-like products, "magic bullets" to prevent or treat diseases, produced great excitement in public and research communities. Discovering biological disease mechanisms and how to intervene on those mechanisms became the almost exclusive focus of spending on research to protect and improve health. The expanding evidence that common habits of living were causing the modern epidemics attracted relatively little attention from the National Institutes of Health and their biomedical constituencies. The medical research community investigated the bodily changes that constituted pathology, and the mechanisms that yielded those end points, rather than the conditions of life that underlay those processes and how to intervene on those larger factors. The micromechanisms of disease intrigued the biological scientists and their efforts were generously supported. Examining living circumstances, how people responded to those circumstances, and how to effect favorable changes in those circumstances found little encouragement.

On the other hand, it seemed obvious that human biology had evolved over the millennia, enabling people's bodies to cope with the world's conditions, for example, certain atmospheric conditions. When the evolved biological limits were exceeded, however, such as by exposure to such new conditions as tobacco smoke, many human bodies could not cope and hence became diseased. Some of us wanted to investigate the social changes that induced such loss of health, rather than to explore how certain chemicals caused lung tissue changes that culminated in cancer. But if it wasn't pursued in a laboratory with glassware or a clinic with patients, the prevailing notion was that it wasn't health research.

The Human Population Laboratory Proposal

Nevertheless, by the late 1950s, success in our morbidity survey studies and the emerging concepts of health and disease causation emboldened us to attempt health measurement using the World Health Organization definition. The 1959 application we submitted to the National Institutes of Health for funding the Human Population Laboratory in Alameda County proposed a planning grant for a project:

1. To assess the health, including physical, mental and social dimensions, of persons living in Alameda County, California;
2. To ascertain whether particular levels in one dimension of health tend to be associated with comparable levels in other dimensions; and
3. To determine relationships of various demographic characteristics and ways of living (including personal habits, familial, cultural, economic and environmental factors) to levels of health.

Our proposal paralleled somewhat two community health studies that were already under way, one in Framingham, Massachusetts, focused on cardiovascular disease (Gordon & Kannel, 1982) and the other in Tecumseh, Michigan, for studying disease more comprehensively. Our concept differed from those two, however, in that we chose to investigate health in a generic sense, rather than in disease-specific terms, and to study it in a modern urban community—the kind of place where an increasing proportion of the population were living—rather than in a relatively small community like Framingham or Tecumseh. Alameda County's demography was similar to the U.S. population, though not statistically representative of it.

Because our application did not match the mission and composition of any already established scientific review body, the NIH assembled a special 15-person group to examine our proposal's merit as a basis for the funding decision. Only a relatively few people were working in the general sociomedical field and probing outside the usual NIH biomedical confines, so practically all those selected knew me on a first-name basis. As the Principal Investigator I invited the visiting team, the accompanying NIH staff, and our HPL group to a highly enjoyable party at my home the evening preceding the review. That event, consistent with a fairly common practice then, would now be frowned upon as an unacceptable effort to influence the group. What happened in the review of our proposal indicates the influence that such cronyism and hospitality then exerted. For the next two days the review team poked into every aspect of the project, after which they engaged in a half-day closed-session deliberation. At the conclusion of that session the chairman (we didn't have chairpersons in those days) announced to me the unanimous decision: absolute rejection. No one favored approval or even suggested revisions that might make our proposal acceptable. Because it was simply too far beyond what the NIH was supposed to do, even in the minds of my friends and colleagues, the panel pronounced the project dead.

That result severely disappointed us, of course, the more so because the application culminated our efforts over several years, and we had been reasonably optimistic.

A few months later, while I was still suffering from the rejection and wondering how to proceed, a telephone call from Harold Dorn surprised me. A National Cancer Institute senior statistician-epidemiologist, who had earlier expressed interest in both our cancer investigations and our health survey methodological studies, Dorn suggested another review. I readily accepted that proposal, of course, though without much hope. For that second evaluation Dorn came with Lowell Reed, the distinguished biostatistician at Johns Hopkins University, as well as its Public Health School Dean and subsequently President of the University, who had known me in the Truman Health Commission work; and Chancellor Gustafson of the University of Nebraska. The three of them spent a half-day with us examining the proposal and then strongly recommended approval.

With NIH funds awarded after that unusual decision-making process we plunged into establishing the Human Population Laboratory which has now been supported by NIH funding steadily for more than four decades. Our major initial efforts consisted of developing the necessary relationships within the Department and the Alameda County community, and outlining our next steps. By 1962 we had received approval for a five-year project with three primary aims:

1. to explore and develop a new concept of health and to construct and test appropriate indices of measurement for this concept;
2. to define and solve certain methodological problems such as optimal design for methods of data collection, validity, reliability, and migration;
3. to provide professional assistance in sampling, data collection, and other aspects of survey research to other units in the Department in the conduct of their epidemiologic studies.

Conceptual Issues

Grasping the World Health Organization definition of health more fully and converting it into operational terms was our central conceptual problem in the Human Population Laboratory. Besides examining health in its generic sense we considered various life situations, for example, "slum-man": the single, homeless, middle-aged man in large cities. Called alcoholic, unemployable, psychotic, and recalcitrant, he is all too familiar in the inner parts of metropolitan communities. His morbidity and mortality rates are high from acute alcoholism, cirrhosis of the liver, tuberculosis, "accidents," and suicide. What appears on his death certificate, however, is probably not too important. Determining whether tubercle bacilli, high blood alcohol or some other drug, liver fibrosis, or a bullet finally ends his life will not advance our understanding much. We need to examine his situation in broader terms—physically, psychologically, and socially—because it is obviously his whole life pattern that leads to an extremely pathological state. If slum-man lies at one end of the health spectrum, then perhaps "university-man" occupies the other end; he will live nearly twice as long and largely free of slum-man's problems. One exhibits very poor and the other very good health, both arising largely from their living situations.

At any one time every person's health may be delineated as somewhere on each of three health spectra: physical, mental and social well-being. Perhaps, we thought, those points could be ascertained for persons representing a population. Considerations such as the seeming inadequacy of prevailing medical theory to explain some significant health problems; recognition that one health condition may result from many factors, and that one factor may result in several ailments; how different health conditions interrelate; the inappropriateness of current diagnostic categories for understanding important modern health problems; emerging knowledge connecting complex social states to several diseases; the evident need to step back from present disease-oriented epidemiology and examine what can be learned by considering health broadly in relation to conditions of life were some of the issues we investigated during early work in the Human Population Laboratory.

Von Bertalanffy, Selye, and Dubos as well as scholars in the epidemiologic tradition such as Cassel, Dorn, Reed, and Lilienfeld greatly influenced our thinking in the Human Population Laboratory. Using the World Health Organization definition, we decided to measure an individual's health along the three health spectra (Belloc, Breslow, & Hochstim, 1971; Berkman, 1971; Renne, 1974) to ascertain what influenced where individuals landed on a health spectrum, and to regard death as one end of the spectrum. Using this overall conceptual framework in a baseline study, we tested our approach to physical, mental, and social well-being separately, but with a view to their somehow being ultimately combined.

Methodological Issues

Even while these conceptual matters were being thrashed out in staff discussions, we started the project's methodological work. How would the individuals be selected to represent Alameda County's adult population? What data would be collected to place each individual somewhere on the three spectra of health? How could we best assure reliability and validity of the data?

Achieving credible health measurement by population surveys required establishing that people could and would report health and health-related information about themselves accurately. The Hagerstown, San Jose, and other studies had provided some evidence for the validity of such data, but we believed that further corroboration would be helpful. Also, was the sample selection process reliable enough in revealing the general population's characteristics accurately? Another key issue was the cost of data collection because most previous health survey information had been obtained through personal interviews, a relatively expensive procedure. Could less costly methods (e.g., telephone interviews or self-administered questionnaires) yield essentially the same quality of information? Further, because we wanted to track people's health throughout the remaining period of life, could we establish and maintain effective contact with respondents and thus ensure their providing ongoing information periodically? Such methodological research occupied us during 1960–1965, when we had to satisfy ourselves as well as the NIH bodies reviewing our work concerning several particular questions:

1. Will people cooperate in using a long mail questionnaire containing many personal questions?
2. If other data collection methods do not suffice, is personal interview follow-up worth the cost?
3. How much bias results from the failure of some people to complete the designated sample even with intensive follow-up?
4. How much of an original sample of people can be traced for several years and then induced to participate in a second survey? Will so many be lost that attenuation severely biases the sample?
5. What can we learn about the validity of the responses? To what extend do they represent reality?
6. How consistently do people respond to the same questions in a health survey? How reliable are their answers?

That preliminary work resulted in several publications and unpublished reports (Hochstim, 1963, 1964, 1967, 1970). The studies disclosed some fascinating things. For example, when personally interviewed, women reported consuming a certain amount of alcohol; the identical questions posed in a telephone interview indicated larger consumption; and a written questionnaire completed by a similar sample revealed an even greater amount. Evidently, for a socially sensitive question like alcohol consumption, the more impersonal the inquiry the more, and presumably the more accurate, social deviance is reported. We also found, contrary to prevailing opinion, that health and health-related data obtained by self-report in written questionnaire format were essentially similar in quality to those secured by telephone or personal interview— and much less expensive to collect. The three strategies yielded return rates varying only from 88 to 93 percent, and nonresponse to 61 questionnaire items varied only from 0.9 to 1.9 percent. Moreover, responses to demographic items were very similar to the 1960 census findings for Alameda County. Such studies and cost effectiveness, which we also ascertained, strongly favored the self-administered questionnaire for collecting health and related information from study subjects.

Findings indicated highly satisfactory reliability (i.e., consistency of individuals' responses to the same questions posed a second time) and validity (i.e., consistency of responses with some other, in this case medical, determination of phenomena as the criterion). For example, in one study 96 percent of the original questionnaire responses to 33 questions concerning specific physical problems were consistently repeated on a second form of the questionnaire. A check with medical records of 739 Kaiser Health Plan patients in the study showed higher than 95 percent agreement on chronic disabilities, chronic conditions, and impairments; and 84 percent on symptoms. My colleagues in the HPL published such data, which other investigators using survey methods for health research valued highly.

We decided that an area probability sample would be the most feasible way of representing Alameda County's adult population, provided we could achieve a satisfactory response rate. Individuals would be selected through a household sampling frame representing all noninstitutionalized County residents over 20 years of age. Our studies encompassing validity, reliability, and economic considerations led us to select a mail questionnaire as the key data collection instrument.

After these decisions we proceeded with a field test in preparation for the Baseline Study. Approximately 2,000 households in Alameda County, one per 150 residences, were randomly chosen and their occupants determined. Counting of the inhabitants was completed in 97 percent of the occupied households, and 90 percent of the enumerated sample completed the questionnaire. The field test entailed using a primary method of data collection: mail, telephone, or personal interview, supplemented by callbacks and other means as necessary to obtain maximum response. It confirmed what we had been learning from our previous methodological work, not only about the response rates but also their completeness, cost, reliability, and validity. Analysis showed that the three strategies yielded practically the same data, quantitatively and qualitatively (Hochstim, 1967). The mail strategy, however, was the most economical. We adopted it for the Human Population Laboratory studies, and it also encouraged the U.S. Bureau of the Census to explore and ultimately use it for collecting certain data in the 1970 census.

Baseline HPL Study and Initial Findings

We devoted several years to determining the content and format of a questionnaire and pilot-testing it for assembling data about people's demographic characteristics; their health status, defined as physical, mental, and social well-being; and their behavioral patterns that might relate to their health status. Questions about demography were fairly standard: age, sex, race, education, and income level. While others at the time were also exploring health measurement in the generic sense, we decided to follow explicitly the WHO concept by measuring physical, mental, and social well-being separately, adopting all three of these domains as the paradigm for measuring health as a whole (Belloc et al., 1971; Berkman, 1971; Renne, 1974). Reaching agreement on details required long HPL staff discussions as well as extensive literature review concerning how people could be categorized on each health dimension along a spectrum from very poor to excellent, and how to select items and phrase questions for the questionnaire.

Our sampling scheme for what we called the Baseline Study (which became the first step in the major long-term investigation), yielded 8,267 persons over 20 years of age representing Alameda County's adult population in 1965. The mail strategy for data collection, which included repeated letters and, ultimately, personal interviews for maximum response, produced 6,928 completed questionnaires.

For physical health we adopted the following health status categories shown in Table 5; the proportions of Alameda County's population that the Baseline Study actually found in each category are also shown. The findings were strongly consistent with what was generally recognized about the relationship of physical health to demographic characteristics; for example, physical health status was lower with increasing age, less income, and being separated, divorced, or widowed.

TABLE 5   Measurement of Physical Well-Being

Percent in Category		Categories of Physical Well-Being
7%	1.	Severe disability: trouble with feeding, dressing, climbing stairs, getting outdoors, or inability to work for six months or longer
8%	2.	Lesser disability: decreasing hours, changing type of work, or cutting down on other activities for six months or longer
9%	3.	No such disability but during the past 12 months two or more chronic conditions or impairments, selected from a list of 18 presented on the questionnaire
19%	4.	Only one such impairment or chronic condition
28%	5.	No such disability, impairment, or chronic condition but one or more symptoms selected from a list presented on the questionnaire (including tightness in chest, back pain)
23%	6.	None of the above but low to medium energy level—fewer than 3 "high energy" answers to questions
6%	7.	None of the above and high energy level—at least 3 "high energy" answers

Measurement of mental well-being posed greater difficulty than physical well-being did. After examining several mental health indices that had appeared in the literature, we settled on a relatively simple, eight-item test aimed at ascertaining a person's psychological well-being. A classic mental health investigation conducted in New York City, the Midtown Manhattan Mental Health study, had indirectly and provisionally validated a very similar instrument; its brevity also enhanced its desirability. The questions included five negative feelings:

- very lonely or remote from other people
- depressed or very unhappy
- bored
- so restless you couldn't sit for long in a chair
- vaguely uneasy about something without knowing why

and three positive feelings:

- on top of the world
- particularly excited or interested in something
- pleased about having accomplished something

Responses were then weighted according to whether people reported experiencing these feelings "never," "sometimes," or "often," and assembled to indicate their mental health. We used a seven-category spectrum on which to array the Alameda County population's mental health. Findings revealed that demographic distribution of mental health in the HPL study group also paralleled what had already become fairly well established in the literature: it was poorer among young people and the elderly, whereas those 45 to 74 years of age showed generally better mental health, and it showed quite steady improvement with level of income and education. Married people enjoyed better mental health than those who were never married or were separated, divorced, or widowed. The findings also confirmed a positive association between physical and mental health status when taking gender, age, and income into account.

Social well-being is commonly envisaged as a community's income level, education, housing, and other requisites for living, and it is often associated with what is generally regarded as health promotion. For example, the great medical and public health historian, Henry Sigerist, remarked that "health is promoted by providing a decent standard of living, good labor conditions, education, physical culture, means of rest and recreation" (Sigerist, 1943). Data that contrast health in industrialized vs. developing nations or in Beverly Hills vs. Harlem exemplify that notion of social well-being.

In the HPL, however, we considered social well-being to be a third dimension of a person's health, an attribute of individuals rather than an attribute of communities. We defined social well-being as how closely an individual is attached to his or her social milieu. That meant determining a person's employability (as in educational achievement, occupational status, and job experience), marital satisfaction, if married, sociability (i.e., number of close friends and relatives), and community involvement (e.g., church attendance, organizational memberships, and political activity). Thus, a socially healthy individual is a functioning community member who meets the cultural expectations of a particular community, in our case, Alameda County in 1965. We found that the population could be distributed along a social health spectrum, this time consisting of nine categories for married persons and six for unmarried, roughly paralleling the physical and mental health domains. Findings revealed strong associations between social health status and both physical and mental health.

Although crude in many respects, the effort did seem to demonstrate that measuring health in the WHO sense was feasible. Rather than simply counting people as diseased or healthy, the Human Population Laboratory counted every person as having a certain degree of health, ranging from excellent to very poor, in each of the three domains. We published data describing the population's health in these terms, relating it to demographic characteristics such as age, gender, income, and educational level, and thus we achieved a significant original aim of the HPL (Breslow, 1972).

Health and Ways of Living

Because we intended the HPL to be a resource not only for measuring health but also for investigating the relationship of health to the ways people lived, we examined factors that might influence health, with attention first to the physical well-being dimension. We hypothesized that a favorable place on the physical health spectrum would be associated with the following: (1) not smoking, (2) drinking little, if any, alcohol, (3) maintaining moderate weight, (4) being physically active, (5) sleeping seven to eight hours a night, (6) regular meals (not just snacking), and (7) eating breakfast. We hypothesized that the extent to which one followed these seven habits were important aspects of lifestyle related to physical health.

Results disclosed that at every age from 20 to 75 years (persons in the HPL sample over 75 were too few for stable computation) people who followed all seven good health habits experienced better physical health status, as we had measured it, than those who followed six; six better than five, and so on (Belloc & Breslow, 1972). In fact, middle-aged persons who followed all seven had about the same physical health status as those 30 years younger who followed only zero to two, and those following six about the same as persons 25 years younger who followed only zero to two.

These findings were so striking that when my colleagues presented them to me I thought they were playing some prank. However, the findings were real; each of the seven practices appeared independently associated with physical health status. Some were more strongly correlated than others, but as the pattern of habits substantially exceeded the strength of any one or two we emphasized the entire pattern in our reports. Rather than single habits we would note their number as the important variable.

We recognized, of course, that our physical health status measure involved a new approach to determining that status and thus might not impress those who wanted a more generally accepted measure as the basis for assessing lifestyle's impact on health. We therefore immediately decided to follow the sample population's mortality; counting subsequent deaths would be more convincing of lifestyle's relevance to health than simply finding a concurrent association between physical health status, as we measured it, and the habits. Repeated analyses of the deaths among the 7,000 persons in the Baseline Study for more than three decades have demonstrated that adherence to the seven health practices strongly and consistently affects the irrefutable end point, death. Even the first mortality check, five and a half years after the study's start, disclosed that 45-year old men who followed zero to three health practices had a further longevity of only 67 years; four to five health practices, 73 years; and six to seven health practices, 78 years. The data for women showed a similar relationship (Belloc, 1973). That 11-year male longevity difference, dependent on health practices, is approximately twice the increase in longevity among American men aged 45 years during the seven decades (1900–1970) when substantial economic advances and improvements in surgery, chemotherapy, and the like occurred. Under age 45, of course, medical services such as childhood vaccinations and chemotherapy have exerted a great influence on premature mortality during the early years of life. As most Americans now live and want good health well beyond age 45, however, the significance of health habits for longevity among people over that age becomes apparent. Although life extension is commonly attributed to medical services, how one lives appears to be a greater influence on longevity, particularly during life's second half.

The early findings thus encouraged us to follow the 1965 Alameda County cohort meticulously by maintaining contact with survivors and their relatives as well as checking state and national death rosters. Meanwhile, surveys have been conducted among the cohort survivors every six to nine years with essentially the same information being collected each time so as to permit tracking of health status, health habits, and other characteristics. Hence, it has been possible to conduct extensive analyses of health status and its predictors, based on the periodically assembled longitudinal data on the 1965 cohort representing the Alameda County general population over 20 years of age.

One analysis has shown that the extent to which people follow the health practices predicts physical disability as strongly as it predicts mortality, taking into account age, gender, baseline physical health status, and social network index. Thus, people with good health habits not only live substantially longer, but they do so with substantially less disability than people with poor health habits (see Figures 1 and 2).

Further Results

In addition to hundreds of papers using the findings, the data have served as the basis for more than a dozen doctoral dissertations. One,

HEALTH PRACTICES AND DISABILITIES

Number of Good Health Practices

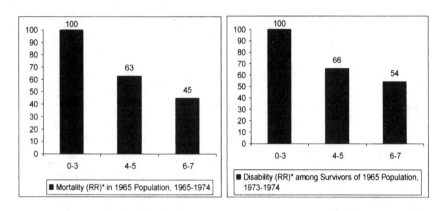

FIGURE 1. Mortality, disability, and health practices among 1965 adult residents of Alameda County, California, 1965–1974. *Adjusted for age, physical health status, and social network in 1965 and gender.

Number of Good Health Practices

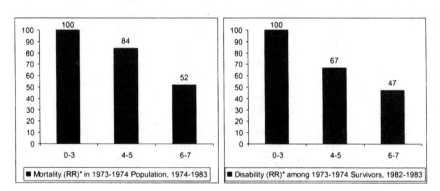

FIGURE 2. Mortality, disability, and health practices among 1973–1974 survivors of Alameda County, California, 1982–1983. *Adjusted for age, physical health status, and social network index in 1972–1973 and gender.

Source: "Health Practice and Disability: Some Evidence from Alameda County," by L. Breslow and N. Breslow, 1993, *Preventive Medicine, 22,* pp. 86–95.

for example, that was based on certain details from the HPL social well-being index to form a measure of social network, showed that a stronger social network predicted lower mortality, roughly paralleling the influence of the seven health practices (Berkman & Syme, 1979).

The findings have also stimulated many replications. As noted earlier, United States Public Health Service and Census Bureau personnel, who developed the National Health Interview Survey, participated in the early Human Population Laboratory work and thereby added to their own health survey experience. After the Alameda County studies showed how significantly the seven health habits affect health, the National Health Interview Survey incorporated very similar questions into the 1977 national survey, and again in 1983, with results similar to those in Alameda County. The 1979 National Survey of Personal Health Practices and Consequences conducted by the National Center for Health Statistics essentially replicated the Alameda County design on a national scale. Periodic measures of national health-related habit trends in the Behavioral Risk-Factor Surveillance System (BRFSS) have subsequently become standard practice in the United States.

In addition to these national replications, similar surveys have been conducted in several states, including Michigan in 1978 and Wisconsin in 1986, as well as in some local communities, branches of the United States Armed Services, and foreign countries. Recognition of the HPL's significance for health measurement probably led to my being appointed chair of the National Committee on Health Statistics for 1979–1981.

Although in 1968 I left the California Department of Public Health, where the Human Population Laboratory was developed and has continued, I have remained in touch with its operations. It has been one of my most satisfying career experiences, including initiating the work, seeing the product, and observing its impact.

RECENT THOUGHTS

Although in the HPL we emphasized the spectrum concept of health ranging over several points—from severe disability to absence of disability, then chronic conditions, symptoms, up to a high level of energy—most attention has gone to people at the poorer health part of the spectrum. Now, however, having observed the long and substantial trend toward better health, my interest has begun to focus not only on the WHO original concept of well-being but on the (WHO) Ottawa Charter's more advanced notion of health as a "resource for living" and as "capacity . . . to realize aspirations and satisfy needs."

That idea, what some call "positive" health, appears to be gradually spreading, and the time may be arriving to consider how that aspect of health can be measured. If one considers it to be "a resource for living," then it may be measured as competence in various features of life, roughly outlined as follows:

Measurement of Health

1. Immunologic (e.g., immunity to influenza and pneumonia)
2. Anatomic (e.g., height–weight ratio (BMI)
3. Physiologic (e.g., walk one-half mile)
4. Chemical (e.g., blood cholesterol, including LDL and HDL)
5. Psychic (e.g., memory)
6. Social (e.g., contact with relatives and friends)

This perhaps too-crudely-expressed concept predicts a next step in health measurement. We do need to get beyond the mere avoidance of disease and disability and move toward extending the healthier part of the spectrum. That is where much emphasis will be placed in future efforts for health improvement.

Tobacco Control 7

Tobacco use in the form of cigarettes has been the greatest pestilence in the United States during the twentieth century because of its role in causing major diseases. Tobacco smoking is linked most prominently to lung cancer, probably because it causes 80–90 percent of such cases which account for about one-twelfth of all deaths. The habit, however, also contributes substantially to other cancers as well as to coronary heart disease and chronic obstructive lung disease. Toward the end of the century experts estimated smoking to be responsible for one-fifth of all deaths (McGinnis & Forge, 1993). In every year between 1968 and 1988 it was responsible for about as many deaths in the United States as all those Americans who died in war during the twentieth century (Centers for Disease Control, 1989). Its toll still exceeds 400,000 deaths annually. Attacking it during the second half of the twentieth century became a prominent feature of the second public health revolution, that is, against the noncommunicable diseases. Even though progress against tobacco has been accelerating, at the start of the twenty-first century its destructive effects are still extensive in this country and are spreading around the world.

The adult per capita consumption of cigarettes in the United States began to rise during the first decade of the twentieth century when it was less than 100 packages of cigarettes annually per 1,000 population. It began a steep rise after the first World War to reach about 800 in 1920, and continued to more than 1,000 in 1930; thereafter, the rate approximately doubled during the 1930s and again in the 1940s (Warner, 1985). Roughly paralleling that increase but about twenty-five years later, lung cancer deaths rose from being very low the first three decades of the century, nearly doubling in the 1930s, and again in the 1940s. The increase continued from 15 deaths per 100,000 in 1950 to 37 in 1970, reaching a peak of 59 in 1990 (National Center for Health Statistics, 2003).

Tobacco use has had a long history in North America. Sixteenth-century European explorers discovered that the Native Americans smoked it, especially on ceremonial occasions such as when taking up the "peace pipe." The colonists from Europe brought tobacco use back to their home countries, where it spread slowly, and male immigrants to America later adopted smoking. During the nineteenth century American smokers commonly hand-wrapped tobacco in a thin paper to make cigarettes. I recall as a youngster in the early 1920s seeing older men still "rolling their own," using tobacco from tin cans and thin papers designed for the purpose. Manufactured cigarettes, however, were already becoming the dominant pattern of tobacco consumption by the 1920s.

As early as 1881 industrial technology had made possible the mechanical manufacturing and packaging of cigarettes. Convenience encouraged their mass consumption and marketing then became a major feature of the industry, which expanded rapidly after World War I. The "dough-boys," becoming addicted to nicotine by cigarettes that were distributed with their Army rations in France, returned home and popularized the product among American males generally. Even some females, particularly those known as "flappers" in the 1920s, started smoking cigarettes, but American women in large numbers started the habit only 20 years later when they entered World War II industry workplaces. Early opposition to tobacco use came mainly from the Seventh-Day Adventist movement and the Women's Christian Temperance Union (WCTU), which campaigned against it on moral and hygienic grounds.

Indicative of how popular smoking had become, as an 8-year-old, I joined a group of kids wanting to appear grown up and thus we decided to smoke. On Saturday mornings in the fall a few of us would buy corn-cob pipes (stem and cup, five cents each) at the store on the edge of town as we walked toward the baseball park. On the way there we filled our pockets with brown corn silk that we took from the ends of the ripe corn that was growing across the fence along the road. In the stadium the one who had been assigned the task that day would produce a box of big matches that he had sneaked from his family kitchen. Then we would "light up and smoke." Our substitute for tobacco did not burn very well, however, and each session lasted only until we had finished the matches. As an adolescent, I tried several brands of cigarettes, but all of them hurt my throat, so I promptly quit. Later, as a medical intern, not being able to tolerate cigarettes but really wanting to be a smoker,

I tried a long-stem pipe, which also proved unsatisfying, so I abandoned smoking without ever becoming addicted.

My first encounter with the problem of smoking and health came in 1946, shortly after I began work in the California Department of Public Health. In my criticism of a health pamphlet prepared by the State Department of Education, which had been referred to me for "health expert" review, I literally blue-penciled a statement that cigarette smoking was harmful to health because at that time I believed that the claim lacked evidence. A few physicians had voiced the idea that it injured health, including Alton Ochsner and Michael DeBakey, surgeons who asserted that it caused lung cancer (Ochsner & DeBakey, 1941). Such views, however, were based on anecdotal accounts, not on scientifically assembled and interpreted facts. The major opposition to cigarettes then seemed based on moralistic grounds, and I rejected such assertions.

STUDIES OF SMOKING AND HEALTH

A short time later, however, I joined other epidemiologists in recognizing the increasing lung cancer incidence and in seeking its cause. The epidemic was occurring over decades rather than weeks, as was true of most epidemics with which we were familiar. Actually, as early as 1938, Pearl had found that smoking was "statistically associated with an impairment of life duration" (Pearl, 1938, p. 216). That finding, however, attracted little attention. Evarts Graham, who in 1933 first removed a cancerous lung, was among those thoracic surgeons who were suggesting that cigarette smoking was causing the disease. In 1952, when he served on President Truman's Health Commission for which I was the Study Director, Graham told me that frequently observing tobacco-stained fingers on his lung cancer patients' hands attracted him to the idea. Graham himself had such fingers and ultimately died of lung cancer. Those rare individuals in the medical or scientific communities who claimed an adverse health effect nonetheless could adduce little or no evidence for their assertions, and gained practically no attention. The main opposition to smoking continued to take a moralistic form.

In the late 1940s Graham encouraged a medical student in St. Louis, Ernst Wynder, to co-investigate the cigarette-lung cancer hypothesis (Wynder & Graham, 1950). Wynder initiated a case/control study, which meant interviewing lung cancer patients and people with similar personal characteristics such as age, gender, and hospital confinement (but not having lung cancer) in order to contrast their cigarette smoking practices. Knowing about our chronic disease program, Wynder sought my help in obtaining entry to San Francisco Bay Area hospitals for his interviews. I was quite skeptical of Wynder's hypothesis; our Bureau of Chronic Disease group was just then deeply engaged in studies to ascertain occupational factors in the disease, following the lead of Wilhelm Hueper in the U.S. Public Health Service (Breslow, 1955a). Hueper had come from Germany, where several investigators had identified certain occupational exposures as causing cancer. His idea that occupational factors were causing the lung cancer epidemic impressed me not only because of the European evidence he brought with him, but also because the epidemic was then affecting only men (who might have significant occupational exposure). We did identify in our studies several types of work that carried a high risk for the disease, including lead, zinc, and copper mining in the Colorado plateau. We later realized that the patients had been exposed to radon there, and possibly might even have mined radium for our atomic bombs. (Occupational factors in lung cancer have unfortunately not received the attention they deserve. For example, they may account in part for the higher mortality rate from that disease among Africa-American men than among whites, a discrepancy not yet clearly delineated.)

I agreed to assist Wynder in his study and sent a young colleague of mine along with him to the hospitals that had agreed to allow their patients to participate. My colleague returned with an alarming tale that the young medical student was not selecting patients as controls in any systematic manner and might thereby be generating a considerable bias. Also, his interviewing seemed quite erratic in that he formulated his questions to the patients in various ways rather than in a standard protocol. Horrified that I had been involved in such activity, I resolved that we would carry out a proper study. We were able to do so simply by adding a few questions about smoking to our then current investigation of occupational factors in the disease.

Greatly surprising to us, our findings very closely approximated Wynder's. Occupational factors apparently did cause some cases, but tobacco clearly was the overwhelming etiological agent of the disease. Our repeat investigation yielded the same results as Wynder obtained probably because the association between smoking and lung cancer was so strong that whether research methods were crude or refined, they would disclose it. Cigarette smokers appeared to have about ten times the risk of non-smokers.

Such early epidemiological studies of the problem conducted by dozens of investigators in the United States consisted of case/control or retrospective investigations in which one simply contrasted the extent of cigarette smoking among lung cancer cases with that among controls. Although the fact that many such studies yielded essentially the same results about the role of smoking was impressive, obviously more convincing evidence would come from a cohort or prospective type of investigation. In the latter a population is first defined, presumably no members of which have lung cancer, and cigarette smoking habits are ascertained for all members. Follow-up observation of the entire cohort then determines which members develop lung cancer (and/or other diseases), and analysis of the data shows the quantitative relationship between smoking and the disease. Because cigarette smoking then would clearly precede the disease occurrence, the statistical estimation of relative risk would be more straightforward than in the case/control studies.

Starting in the late 1940s and early 1950s, several epidemiologists in the U.S. and the U.K. initiated prospective studies. The earliest reported was that of Richard Doll and Bradford Hill, who examined health consequences of cigarette smoking among British physicians (Doll & Hill, 1952). One important advantage of prospective studies on cigarette smoking is that one can ascertain its relationship to total mortality and to all major specific diseases to which deaths in the observed population may be attributed. Thus, in addition to lung cancer, we learned about smoking's causation of coronary heart disease, emphysema, and other conditions that result in considerable morbidity and mortality.

EXTENDING THE CONVICTION THAT SMOKING DAMAGES HEALTH

Epidemiologists, especially those engaged in the studies of smoking and health, had been almost universally convinced in the early 1950s that cigarette smoking was causing the lung cancer epidemic.

With the major evidence essentially all gathered and analyzed by the mid-1950s, epidemiologists launched the struggle to convince others in the medical scientific community, those in health policy positions, and the general public that cigarette smoking caused lung cancer. In that effort and in the preceding research phase these epidemiologists became well-acquainted with each other, and from our various positions we vigorously espoused the findings from our studies: Richard Doll, who with Bradford Hill had conducted the prospective study among British physicians, led the world-wide effort; E. Cyler Hammond and Daniel Horn, sponsored by the American Cancer Society, helped develop that important organization's policy (Hammond & Horn, 1958); Wynder and I concentrated on the American preventive medicine and public health communities.

The tobacco companies fought intensely against the research results and their implications. Among many other public relations, lobbying, and advertising efforts, the industry established its own Tobacco Research Council (TRC) in order to counter the growing scientific conclusions and the likelihood that they would become the basis for policy. The tobacco companies recruited several scientists to work for the TRC and expended considerable monies publicizing its statements. The industry view actually penetrated many agencies in all layers of government, and during the middle and late 1950s even the American Cancer Society's Board of Directors, where laymen reflecting corporate interests held up the Society's action against smoking for several years, despite advocacy of such efforts by the members with medical and scientific backgrounds (Breslow et al., 1977). Years later, when the evidence became overwhelming, the American Cancer Society began playing a vigorous anti-smoking role.

The scientific debate chiefly concerned the question of whether any research other than an experiment could prove a causal connection. The conviction that only an actual experiment could provide satisfactory evidence, which had evolved during the research that proved the causation of microbial diseases, continued to dominate the scientific community's thinking. Obviously, however, a definitive experimental approach to the lung cancer matter would have involved subjecting humans to smoking and thus was utterly impossible in the light of available knowledge. Therefore, it was necessary to rely on observational data, but some scientists continued to insist strongly that only experimental data were sufficient to prove causation.

It was not until 1959 that the Surgeon General of the Public Health Service, declared "the weight of the evidence . . . implicates smoking as the principal etiological factor in the increasing incidence of lung cancer" (Burney, 1959). That statement came after considerable research as well as rhetoric had been devoted to elucidating the matter.

IMPACT OF THE SURGEON-GENERAL'S REPORT

Consensus was steadily emerging as the evidence accumulated. The subsequent Surgeon General, Luther Terry, appointed an expert committee, none of whose members had taken a public position and all of whom were approved by the tobacco industry, to review the evidence. In 1964, that committee's Report, based on animal, autopsy, and (principally) epidemiological studies, stated that "cigarette smoking is causally related to lung cancer in men; the magnitude of the cigarette smoking effect far outweighs all other factors. The data for women, though less extensive, points in the same direction" (Surgeon General's Advisory Committee,

1964, p. 37). That Surgeon General's statement on the issue placed great emphasis on the prospective studies, identifying seven as the most significant in proving the causal relationship to lung cancer. Included in that group were two of our California prospective investigations. The Report essentially ended the scientific debate and called for unspecified "remedial action." The Tobacco Research Council did manage after 1964 to support a few scientists in conducting and publishing works alleging doubt about the link, but they carried rapidly diminishing weight.

To my mind, moreover, the Surgeon General's Report on Smoking and Health elucidated a related issue that was highly important for health advancement, namely, how to determine proof of causality from observational data. The Report stated that "statistical methods cannot establish proof of a causal relationship in an association. The causal significance of an association is a matter of judgment . . . [for which] . . . a number of criteria must be utilized, no one of which is an all-sufficient basis for judgment. These criteria include: (a) the consistency of the association, (b) the strength of the association, (c) the specificity of the association, (d) the temporal relationship of the association, (e) the coherence of the association" (Surgeon General, p. 20).

By delineating and using these criteria in settling the tobacco/lung cancer issue the Committee greatly advanced epidemiology's role in determining causal factors for the chronic diseases generally. Conceptually, they parallel Koch's procedure for determining the causation of bacterial diseases and should be utilized much more explicitly and widely than they have been thus far.

SHIFT TO THE SOCIOPOLITICAL SCENE

After 1964 the tobacco-health battle shifted from the scientific to the sociopolitical scene. The tobacco industry's mega-millions supported lobbying and political campaigns as well as cigarette advertising. That expenditure was designed to entice new cigarette buyers, and to convince legislators that they should avoid action that would negatively affect tobacco consumption. Subsequent disclosures revealed how the industry had concealed its own evidence of harm, especially nicotine addictiveness, and how industry spokespersons had lied about that knowledge, even to Congress (Glantz et al., 1996).

Meanwhile, the campaign against tobacco expanded. For example, attorney John Banzhof III successfully petitioned the Federal Communications Commission to obtain equal media time for anti-cigarette messages. Individuals and local, state, and national organizations, including the American Cancer Society, the American Lung Association, and the American Heart Association, joined the tobacco fray.

Like many others, I began advocating tobacco control measures—for example, during my 1964–1968 tenure on the American Cancer Society Board of Directors; in various consultant relationships to the National Cancer Institute, including service as chair of the Working Group on Cancer Control in the 1973 National Cancer Program Planning Conference; and in 1982, outlining a public policy for smoking control to include:

1. Restriction of who can smoke (e.g., no one under 18 years of age), and where people can smoke, in order to protect non-smokers
2. Restrictions on advertising cigarettes, to counter the tobacco industry's influence in and through the media
3. More public information, to enlighten people about tobacco's adverse health effects
4. Education, including incorporation of instruction about tobacco products into school curricula
5. Aid to persons who want to quit
6. Taxation to discourage smoking, and other economic measures: for example, developing alternative uses of the land and employment of people now devoted to growing tobacco
7. Opposing international marketing of cigarettes, which is systematically addicting the people of developing nations
8. Research, especially into ways of avoiding smoking
9. Exclusion in public policy of efforts to establish a general prohibition against smoking, which would be a counterproductive measure, and efforts to develop a "safe" cigarette with "low tar," as that had been found to be ineffective in eliminating adverse health effects (Breslow, 1982).

PROPOSITION 99 IN CALIFORNIA

California took an early leadership role in implementing the public health steps that flowed from the research findings on tobacco's effect on health. In 1963 the Department of Public Health, having witnessed a series of presentations culminating in its publication, *Cigarette Smoking and Health*, adopted a resolution calling for a statewide campaign to control cigarette smoking as a hazard to health (California Department of Public Health, 1963). The Governor promptly appointed a Governor's Advisory Committee on Smoking and Health, indicating his strong commitment to consider legislation. That Committee's Report in 1964 recommended a coordinated action program stressing education; community service centers, including cigarette withdrawal clinics; an increased tax on cigarettes to fund the program; and evaluation (Governor's Advisory Committee on Smoking and Health, 1964). In my role as Chief of the Department's Division of Preventive Medical Services and with my strong background in tobacco research, I was active in these programs and led the technical staff for the Governor's Committee; Devra, my future wife, served as Editorial Writer for the Report.

The major voluntary health agencies in California concerned about smoking vigorously sought state legislative action that would aid tobacco control by earmarking revenue from a proposed increased tax on cigarettes, but this and similar endeavors met a legislative stonewall that had obviously been constructed and was being maintained largely by tobacco industry influence, reflecting its huge expenditures in political contributions over the years. As late as May 1987, a proposed increase in the tax on cigarettes did not get a single vote in the legislative committee where it was considered.

Exasperated by such failures, the American Lung Association, the American Cancer Society, the American Heart Association, the Service Employees International Union, the California Medical Associations, and the Planning and Conservation League formed an Anti-Tobacco Coalition, which in 1988 succeeded in passing Proposition 99, thus increasing the tax on a package of cigarettes by twenty-five cents. That initiative, which was really a means of bypassing the Legislature, was approved directly by the electorate approximately 60 to 40 percent. It stipulated that the new tobacco tax revenue would be largely devoted to medical and hospital services, but 20 percent of the total was earmarked for tobacco control. The first year's revenue from the increased tax amounted to a half-billion dollars; that meant about $100 million for tobacco control—a considerable amount in public health budgets.

Proposition 99 required the State Legislature to specify how the tobacco control money would be spent, and a group of us professors in major universities around the state held telephone conferences to prepare a proposal for allocating the funds. Because we knew and respected one another and collectively had considerable knowledge of the subject, it was relatively easy for us to achieve consensus: approximately one-fourth of the anticipated $100 million should go to schools throughout the State, on a population-formula basis; and the same proportion to community health agencies on a project-competitive basis; one-eighth to local health departments and one-eighth to a media campaign; and the remainder to data collection, evaluation, and administration. The group designated me as spokesperson to advocate our plan to the Legislature.

Shortly after our proposal became known, Steve Thompson, Chief of the State Assembly's research office and hence directly responsible to the Speaker, invited me to present it to the principal stake-holders. After a discussion of several hours at a Sacramento conference, which brought together about thirty people representing the several interests and ideas concerning how the money for tobacco control should be used, the group endorsed our proposal and asked an American Lung Association activist, Carolyn Martin, and me to present it to the Legislature. We appeared at a large hearing before the relevant combined committees of the Assembly and Senate. As I was walking up to the table for testimony with a briefcase full of material, someone whom I recognized as highly knowledgeable stopped me in the aisle and whispered that the legislators were already convinced to favor our suggested allocation except for considerable opposition to the media item. He urged me to concentrate on that, and I did so. The hearing ended with an overwhelming vote favoring the entire plan, and the Legislature subsequently appropriated the funds largely as we had proposed. However, it mandated that a relatively small proportion of the 20 percent of the funds for tobacco control be used for augmenting the Child Health Disability Program, a totally separate Departmental program with no relationship to smoking. That provision subtly specified that an increasing proportion of the funds be so diverted over time. We failed to note and naively did not protest that action, which would later disrupt the tobacco control program by taking away its funds.

The legislation also provided for a Tobacco Education Oversight Committee (TEOC) to which the Assembly Speaker appointed me as Vice-Chairman. Our task was to maintain surveillance over the new tobacco education programs in the State Health Services and Education Departments, make suggestions for them, and prepare an annual report and plan. The Committee's master plan in January 1991 outlined a comprehensive program that ultimately included a media campaign; restricting access to tobacco, for example, by forbidding vending machine tobacco sales or distributing free samples; smoke-free workplaces and public buildings; school-based education; resources for aiding cessation of tobacco use; training community activists; and evaluation.

Implementation of Proposition 99 proceeded quite smoothly at first, and we were pleased that California's previous rate of smoking decline actually doubled after its passage and during the early 1990s. The tax increase precipitated an immediate drop in smoking as expected, and the program was definitely extending that decline beyond the price increase effect. In its February 1993 report the TEOC noted that adult Californians' smoking prevalence had declined from 26.7 percent in

1988 to 20.4 percent in 1992, concurrent with a wide scope of related community, media, and school activities. The components all seemed to be working: community agencies of many types mobilized their constituencies for tobacco control projects, hard-hitting media messages were attracting attention, and local health departments and schools inaugurated appropriate actions. The 1993 TEOC report also asserted that the decline in smoking prevalence was on target to reach the goal of 6.5 percent of adults smoking by the end of 1999.

The program stimulated anti-tobacco forces in communities throughout California to take action. This took the form of an aggressive media campaign; education about tobacco in local agencies, neighborhoods, and schools; contests and other events that attracted youngsters' attention and support; and, perhaps most significantly, city and county ordinances to remove cigarette vending machines from places where young people had access to them, and to prohibit smoking in restaurants and other public places. Coupled with "sting" operations against retailers selling cigarettes to minors and growing newspaper editorial support, these local activities greatly accelerated the abatement of smoking. So successful was the program's penetration into local communities that the tobacco industry in 1994 attempted with its own initiative (Proposition 188) to establish State preemption of governmental tobacco control action. Popular support for what was underway in local communities and the progress being made against tobacco use, coupled with growing sophistication of the electorate, resulted in a 70–30 percent defeat of Proposition 188, despite tobacco industry expenditure of $19 million for the proposition against $1 million raised in opposition.

INCREASING DIVERSION OF THE FUNDS BY THE LEGISLATURE AND GOVERNOR AND RESTORATION BY THE COURT

The tobacco industry continued to fight the tobacco control movement ferociously. It not only spent $3.1 million in 1987–1988 to defeat Proposition 99, but, having failed in that endeavor, by 1989–1990 the industry had become a major player in California politics, spending $5.4 million in political contributions, according to the Tobacco Education Oversight Committee in 1993.

Three or four years into the program, however, things turned sour. Tobacco industry contributions to California legislators increased sixfold during the five-year period beginning with the Proposition 99 fight and continued thereafter to reach $4,000 on average to each legislator. As another tactic, they initiated and supported various organizations to claim "Smokers' Rights." They found allies in the Legislature, of course, but also in the State Administration, the California Medical Association, and the California Association of Hospitals and Health Systems. The latter groups had managed to insert into the original legislation the provision that some of the 20 percent of the Proposition 99 cancer control funds be increasingly shunted into medical services, allegedly to enhance physician education of preschool and early elementary school youngsters about tobacco. The total new tax revenues, of course, dropped as consumption declined. Program leaders and supporters had anticipated and welcomed that effect of success, but failed to take effective action about the medical diversion trap until considerable damage had been done. Community organizations, local health departments, and schools had expanded staff to educate people about tobacco's harmful health effects and had undertaken substantial efforts to limit them. Because of the diversion of funds, however, they were forced to reduce their work just as the program was getting strongly underway. Morale was shattered and progress sharply curtailed.

The Child Health and Disability Program leaders in both state and local health departments were using the largesse to expand their services generally, with essentially no attention to tobacco control among the children they served, the vast majority of whom were less than 10 years of age. Physicians "educating" such youngsters about tobacco, of course, seemed useless. Appeals to the Legislature and the Governor on behalf of genuine tobacco control yielded nothing, and the tobacco industry was, no doubt, delighted with the turn of events. By 1994 the Health Education Account was used for tobacco control received only 12 percent of the Proposition 99 revenues rather than the 20 percent specified in the Initiative (Novotny & Siegal, 1996).

The 1993 TEOC Report had called for a stop in funding the Child Health Disability Program from the Health Education Account. With no support for remedial action from the Governor or the Legislature, however, it became necessary for the anti-tobacco forces to seek court action in order to reverse the trend. Those espousing genuine tobacco control filed a suit that required the Legislature to stop deflecting money and follow Proposition 99. In 1995, rejecting arguments of the California Medical Association, the California Association of Hospitals and Health Systems, and state officials that the diversion should be continued, the court ruled in favor of the tobacco control forces, and the disputed funds were thereafter distributed to tobacco control as Proposition 99 had mandated.

Meanwhile, unfortunately, the State diversion of tobacco control monies into medical services had drastically limited the funds for local community activities. The cutbacks in support disrupted carefully developed plans. People engaged in the program became discouraged and demoralization set in; loss of funds also interrupted the state media efforts. The decline in smoking slowed. Even after the judicial ruling that reinstated the tobacco control funds to their legal purpose as established by Proposition 99, the State health administration in the mid 1990s failed to support the media program effectively, an action that provoked intense controversy with the TEOC in 1996. Understandable cynicism extended among local officials and community agencies after the major loss of funds for their tobacco control programs.

Despite these adverse events the California tobacco control program has achieved considerable success. Although tobacco industry expenditures in 1989–1990 were approximately three times higher than the expenditures for control, eight times higher in 1994–1995, and ten times higher in 1999–2000; and having reached a plateau in the proportion of smoking (to about 17 percent) among adults in 1994, progress continued. A drop during the late 1990s in the average number of cigarettes smoked per day by everyday smokers from 18 to 15, a one-third decline in the adult per capita consumption, and a fall in the proportion of youths smoking from 11 percent to 6 percent indicated the continuing effect of the program (Evaluation Task Force, California Tobacco Control Program, 2002).

During the 1990s a proportionally greater decline of cigarette smoking occurred in the state than in the country as a whole. Factors in that success probably include direct participation of the State's people in the 60–40 passage of Proposition 99 in 1988 after years when the legislature failed to act on the matter. A substantial cigarette tax increase and the specification that one-fifth of its revenues be used for tobacco control facilitated a serious effort. Legislative action implementing the initiative allocated those funds for a comprehensive program that involved state and local governmental public health and education agencies; community mobilization of numerous organizations to support local education, direct service, and local projects; and a strong state-led media campaign. The breadth and strength of the total effort has apparently changed the general attitude in the state, which formerly tolerated smoking as normal, to antipathy toward it. Owners of restaurants and bars, where smoking is now forbidden, have realized that the injunction has not decreased business. Indoor air is now much cleaner, for which people generally are thankful, and service workers in such places are especially grateful.

The tobacco industry fights every step of the way, using its tremendous resources trying to maintain smoking, which is increasingly becoming limited to people of lower education who seem more vulnerable to billboard advertising and other such appeals. The industry also manages to find allies, especially among legislators whom it rewards well, and, as history shows, various groups, sometimes including medical organizations.

Despite the plateau in the decline of smoking beginning in 1994, which probably reflected the disruption of control efforts, overall results in California give reason for optimism. One may draw several inferences from the experience:

1. A comprehensive tobacco control program should incorporate every means of converting a social milieu that tolerates tobacco use as "normal" to one in which antipathy towards it prevails.
2. Education of young people should emphasize that smoking means they are being exploited by the tobacco industry to the detriment of their health, and that, although some youngsters take up smoking, adults overwhelmingly do not.
3. Maintaining the original broad coalition of program forces generated by Proposition 99—local health departments, schools, and community agencies—has greatly enhanced the effort.
4. An official oversight committee consisting of people outside State government has facilitated keeping the program on track.
5. The tobacco industry never stops the combat. The real battle is not to persuade people individually against tobacco use; it is against the industry itself.
6. Mobilization of community forces and initiative at the local level must be sustained and State preemption avoided.
7. Program stability and continuity must be assured in order to maintain morale and promote steady progress.

In the meantime, of course, following the 1964 Surgeon General's Committee Report, a national program against smoking has been mounting. Efforts by several federal agencies, including the National Cancer Institute for research; The Centers for Disease Control and Prevention for support of tobacco control activities by state and local agencies; and the Federal Trade Commission, which has required health warning labels on cigarette packages, have comprised the effort. The Food and Drug Agency has thus far been thwarted by court action from asserting jurisdiction over tobacco as a drug. In addition to California several other states have passed legislation, some by the initiative process and some directly by the legislatures, to increase tobacco taxes and to allocate the funds raised in that manner to medical services and tobacco control. These state efforts have been somewhat augmented by funds from the Master Tobacco Settlement (see below) which yielded tobacco company monies for the states as a result of the states' suits for damages. Unfortunately, most of these latter funds have simply gone into state coffers to augment revenues from state taxes, rather than into tobacco control.

Still, the success of federal and state activities to curtail tobacco use may be seen in the trend in adult per capita cigarette smoking. It reached a peak nationally in the early 1960s, about eight times higher than it had been just prior to World War I. After increasing steadily to more than 4,000 cigarettes per person per year at the time of the 1964 Surgeon's General Report, consumption has since declined by the end of the century to about 2,000, the same level as that prevailing just before World War II.

OTHER TOBACCO CONTROL ACTIVITIES

A spate of suits by individuals and then states against the tobacco industry seeking compensation for damages caused by tobacco consumption were filed during the 1990s, and some were successful. Although the Proposition 99 program kept my tobacco control energies largely confined to California, I did participate somewhat in relevant legal activities elsewhere. An Ada, Oklahoma, attorney called me as a witness in a suit seeking tobacco company payment of damages for a nineteen-year-old's death from oral cancer, which had originated where he customarily held his tobacco quid since he was twelve. The company's defense included employing a baseball player to walk prominently around the courtroom displaying a tobacco package in his back pocket, and calling as expert witnesses for the defense dozens of biomedical scientists, particularly several pathologists. The jury did not uphold the suit in which the plaintiff's attorney apparently failed to match the legal talent brought in to present the tobacco defense.

When Mississippi filed the first action to indemnify a state for the public expenses that tobacco companies had caused, namely, medical payments for tobacco-induced diseases, I became a witness through a rather circuitous process. The State's Attorney General sought advice from a local attorney and friend who had participated in successful suits against the asbestos industry, and the latter proposed linking up with the Ness-Motley firm in Charleston, South Carolina, which had led the asbestos litigation. That firm agreed to join the Mississippi tobacco suit and contacted its main witness in the asbestos proceedings, Dr. Herbert Abrams. Herb, who had worked with me in the California State Department of Public Health, and recommended me as a tobacco expert. The suit brought Mississippi a substantial sum through an out-of-court settlement, thus making my trial appearance unnecessary. My role involved principally making a deposition and defending it against tobacco industry attorneys. The same firm called me for similar participation in the Florida and Texas cases that ended in the same fashion. Increasingly strong public opinion was aroused by revelations that the tobacco companies had unscrupulously concealed and even denied their own evidence that their products both damaged health and addicted consumers. Success in the first three state suits, and another one in Minnesota, encouraged other states and several local jurisdictions to initiate comparable legal action. That series of blows eventuated in the national Master Tobacco Settlement requiring that the tobacco industry pay more than $200 billion over 25 years to states.

As a member of the Los Angeles County Public Health Commission, which the Board of Supervisors appoints to oversee the County's public health efforts, I participate in reviewing the County's tobacco control program. We learned that the County's Cancer Control budget derived from Proposition 99, which had started at $12 million in 1989–1990, had declined when the state fund diversion occurred; rose again when money came back into the program (up to $20 million one year); but declined sharply in the late 1990s to less than $5 million annually. That meant a second sharp slump in program effort: slashing the program, demoralizing its personnel, and disrupting the dozens of tobacco control projects that community agencies had undertaken.

At the same time the Master Tobacco Settlement funds from the consolidated state suits ($105 million) were coming to the County without any specification for use. Promptly, however, these were committed largely to medical service activities. The Federal government, which five years earlier had bailed the County out of a hospital fiscal crisis, insisted that its support during a second five years would continue only if the County allocated $60 million from the Master Tobacco Settlement toward matching the Federal contribution for medical and related services. That left $45 million for which numerous additional medical service demands confronted the Board of Supervisors: a deteriorating trauma system, deficient mental health services, need to bolster community ambulatory care, and many others. In that milieu I have joined with the major voluntary health organizations, community tobacco control agencies, and elements of the County Department of Health Services to persuade the

Board of Supervisors (thus far without success) that they should utilize Master Tobacco Settlement funds in substantial part to mitigate another continuing County health disaster, this one due to tobacco's effects.

The struggle continues.

Public Health Administration   8

During the first half of the twentieth century, public health agencies grew at federal, state, and local levels, mainly applying the tools that were becoming available for the struggle against the communicable diseases and the health problems of maternity and infancy, and for improvements in sanitation. The U.S. Public Health Service, established in 1912 through expansion of the previous U.S. Public Health and Marine Hospital Service (which had mainly supported the nascent U.S. international commerce by providing medical services to the men who worked on the ships) became the national leader in communicable disease control. Meanwhile the U.S. Children's Bureau, funded by the Sheppard-Towner Act of 1921 and subsequently by Title V of the 1935 Social Security Act, led the nation's maternal and child health program development. Progress during that period entailed developing epidemiological and related laboratory services; immunization programs, whenever effective agents to prevent specific diseases became available; environmental control measures, for example, pasteurization of milk; public health nursing services, especially to families not well prepared for maternal–infant health care; means for combating tuberculosis; and health education.

Public health administration embracing all these activities required community and professional leadership as well as building organizations and managing their functions. It also entailed dealing with other relevant institutions and agencies such as the medical profession, legislative bodies, and governmental executives in various departments. The medical profession's political influence on public health programs and that of legislative bodies at the several levels of government have probably been as important in developing public health programs as the executive branches of government. Although progressive-minded physicians played prominent roles in initiating governmental public health activities, including some clinical services, the dominant elements of the profession essentially regarded all government programs involving medical services as an economic threat to their practices. The two societal arms for health, the one devoted to sick individuals and the other to the health of populations, hence began to diverge.

As Mullan (2000) has pointed out, "Science and politics come face to face in the practice of public health" (p. 702). That happens because public health brings science to the solution of health problems, but the action occurs in the public arena where politics prevails.

During the two decades following Franklin Roosevelt's inauguration as President of the United States in 1933, public health administration gained tremendous maturation, enhancing state, local, and federal health department work. The new president brought in Thomas Parran, who had served as state health officer in New York when Roosevelt was Governor there, to become Surgeon General of the United States Public Health Service (USPHS). Supported by the president as a significant figure in the New Deal, Parran vigorously led the USPHS and the nation out of passively accepting the status quo in public health. Often, with his fearless language—for example, by using the word "syphilis" in a 1936 radio speech—he broke the longstanding taboo on public mention of the disease. Parran was later labeled a communist for espousing national health insurance. His commitment to public health, even if it meant sharply breaking with the medical establishment, may be seen when as incoming Dean of the University of Pittsburgh School of Public Health after he left the Surgeon General's post, he argued against making the School a branch of the University's Medical School, and criticized the medical center for being dominated by faculty who sought mainly arrangements for their private patients, not a true university role.

As Surgeon General, Parran strongly supported Joseph Mountin, a career officer in the USPHS who strenuously advocated a broad view of public health. Mountin's pioneering work included creating the Centers for Disease Control in 1946 (later, "and Prevention" was added to the name) from what had been the Malaria Control in War Areas project during World War II. Later, in the Bureau of State Services, Mountin developed programs for control of water and air pollution, chronic disease, and health of the aging.

In 1939 the USPHS, the Social Security Board, and other agencies were merged into the Federal Security Agency, which has evolved into the Department of Health and Human Services. Other agencies concerned with public health have been created from time to time in various segments of the federal government, for example, the Environmental

Protection Agency, the Occupational Safety and Health Administration, and the Children's Bureau.

Federal health accomplishments in recent decades, however, did not obviate the fundamental responsibility of the states for public health. The U.S. Constitution leaves to the states those powers not specifically allocated to the federal government. Hence the fact that the Constitution does not mention public health, except for foreign quarantine, means that the states have the basic governmental obligation for it. The federal government aids the states in fulfilling their duties by allocating funds and technical support through the interstate commerce provisions of the constitution and other means. Actually, its larger revenue base has permitted the federal government to play a key role in public health.

The national invigoration of public health under Roosevelt-Parran was extended in California by what may be called the Warren-Halverson era when Earl Warren served as Governor and Wilton Halverson as Public Health Director. It was my good fortune to participate in the public health advances that they initiated. During the same time (1946–1967), when I had the opportunity in California to develop a chronic disease control program, engage in international health ventures, and initiate the Human Population Laboratory, I was also involved in state public health administration. That opportunity came about during the supportive political and public health administrative climate that Warren created as Governor, including his appointment of Halverson as Director of Public Health. Warren's contributions as Governor to the state's well-being, beginning in 1943, were recognized as so large and numerous that both Democratic and Republican political parties gave him the nomination for a second term in 1946.

MY EARLY PERSONAL EXPERIENCES IN ADMINISTRATION

My first experience in public health administration occurred during the early 1940s when I served as District Health Officer for the six southeastern counties of Minnesota, which were loosely supervised by the State Health Department's central staff in Minneapolis. My principal responsibility was to coordinate the District staff consisting of a sanitary engineer, a public health nurse, and a secretary (as described in chapter 2). In that environment I came to appreciate the significance of teamwork and especially realized the fundamental contributions being made by the two senior health professionals who were already in the office when I arrived. I learned a great deal about basic public health administration from them, particularly delegation of responsibility to competent colleagues.

The importance of "support from above" for administration (i.e., from higher elements of the organization) impressed me during the Winona syphilis experience (described in chapter 4). Also, in serving the area as health officer I learned how much can be accomplished by working with the local physicians, visiting nurse associations, and others who were part of the communities throughout the southeastern Minnesota counties, and turning to expertise when needed wherever it exists, as in the Kasson epidemic. Those administrative lessons during the early part of my career enriched it mightily.

My military experience had also yielded insight into management, particularly the significance of knowledge about what is being managed as well as skill in the management process itself. I was happy that "Vinegar Joe" Stillwell, my commanding officer in the U.S. Army seventh infantry division had mastered weaponry, military tactics, and logistics in addition to the ability to lead and guide men. I sometimes reflect on that infantry experience when I see the damage that can arise from the belief that "a good manager can manage anything," including public health. That myth has led to many unfortunate outcomes, as when "directors of health" without health experience make decisions on technical matters.

Managing public health effectively requires some specialized knowledge just as commanding an infantry division or conducting a symphony orchestra does. Deficiencies in knowledge in any of these situations can lead to disastrous consequences.

ENTERING A STRONG STATE DEPARTMENT OF PUBLIC HEALTH

Warren and Halverson firmly believed that government should provide excellent public service with justice and fairness to all, and they used their offices as Governor and State Director of Public Health to achieve that goal. Their leadership introduced what in retrospect appears to have been a golden era of social, and especially public health, advances in California. For a good part of that same period the social milieu established by Franklin Roosevelt dominated the national public health scene. One can only wish that the political philosophy to which Roosevelt and Earl Warren adhered during the middle part of the century had continued, instead of being overturned by Reaganism.

Warren not only selected Halverson as Director of Public Health but he also chose professionally competent and effective administrators for welfare, prison, and other public service posts in his administration, delegating responsibility to them for carrying out what he regarded as government's essential social tasks. A spirited group of State Cabinet officers, they demanded excellent staff performance in their departments and created circumstances for its attainment. It was anyone's good fortune to work in that environment. Although loyalty to Warren and his ideology probably served as one criterion for appointment to the top posts, merely being willing to follow a political line was by no means a key factor in being chosen for the State's major public service positions. Professional competence was the predominant criterion. Unfortunately, adherence to a political philosophy did become a major factor in determining who served in some later California State administrations, with considerable damage to morale.

As Director of Public Health beginning in the early 1940s Halverson vigorously followed Warren's leadership in making governmental public health work a professional enterprise. He specifically sought to make California's Department, established in 1870 and the second oldest in the country, the best in the nation. To that end Halverson recruited highly competent people who already were or subsequently became national leaders in their fields to head the State's health programs. Halverson and the two succeeding him as directors of the California State Department of Public Health were each elected to the American Public Health Association presidency.

Besides quality service, Warren's view of public health included a second important element: a strong commitment to equity. With a large family himself he knew what was necessary to obtain medical care. So determined was he to assure appropriate medical services to all people in the State that he introduced and vigorously fought for a State health insurance proposal, a campaign that evoked strong opposition by the medical-profession portion of his constituency. Although unsuccessful in that particular endeavor, Warren strongly supported equity and quality in health services, for example, in the development of maternal and child health care and other clinical services in local public health departments.

Halverson, however, stoutly resisted the Governor's effort to enlist him in the movement for State health insurance because he feared that joining it would jeopardize relations with the medical profession, which he valued as essential to traditional public health work. Nevertheless, knowing that a new member of his staff showed great enthusiasm for the Governor's aim, Halverson did make him (me) available to work on Warren's speeches for State health insurance.

A State Board of Health consisting of outstanding physicians and other knowledgeable citizens provided oversight and support to the Department. Pursuant to State statutes and with the Governor's backing, the Board also had authority to adopt health regulations that carried the force of law. Presentations to the Board by departmental representatives, whether for discussion or formal approval, required careful preparation. A staff member who was reporting usually encountered a searching examination by Board members who did their homework and came prepared with tough questions.

Responsibility of governmental departments for formulating policy, and implementing it when approved, highlighted California public administration in those days. For example, at incoming Governor Pat Brown's request in 1959, the Department of Public Health was mandated to develop and publish standards for safe air quality. Without any further administrative or legislative participation the Department proceeded to do so, and the State Board of Health adopted regulations for air pollution control that were the first in the United States to require decreasing automobile emissions. Nowadays, state and local legislative bodies and the corresponding chief governing officials would likely control and micromanage such a decision with its far-reaching economic and health implications. The California State Board of Health's strength, both in its members and in its authority, bolstered public health programming. It served as substantial protection against political interference by legislators or the Governor's office because the Board operated with considerable autonomy when determining what would be done for public health. In subsequent times, when the Board had been abolished, micromanagement from the Governor's office in California tended to prevail.

Immediately following World War II the California Department of Health was just undergoing structural reorganization into five divisions: Administration, Laboratory Services, Preventive Medical Services, Local Health Services, and Environmental Health Services. The new organization resembled that of most large state health departments at the time, with each Division including several bureaus such as Acute Communicable Disease in the Division of Preventive Medical Services, and Radiation Health in the Division of Environmental Health Services. Several of the California Department program chiefs not only provided stellar services in the state, but they also became national leaders in their fields.

Most elements in the Department were working at the cutting edge of their domains, beyond carrying out more traditional duties. For example, Monroe Eaton in the Virus Laboratory collaborated as a key player in the Rockefeller Foundation-financed project to develop a world-wide influenza tracking system as a step toward avoiding a pandemic like that of 1918–1920. That pandemic had demonstrated the possibility that humankind might be wiped out by some emerging variant of the influenza virus, just as other adverse biologic circumstances had eliminated other species from the earth. The Rockefeller-initiated system continues to the present time for monitoring influenza, augmented by the subsequent development of influenza vaccines used to combat the varying forms of the virus that attack humans. The Virus Laboratory work illustrates how the Department tackled key, long-range public health issues.

When he was appointed State Health Director, Halverson promptly recognized the great administrative talent of Malcolm Merrill, who had been heading the Department's Laboratory Services, so he selected Merrill as his deputy. Believing that in order to function effectively as Deputy-Director of the Department he should broaden his understanding of public health, Merrill enrolled at the U.C. Berkeley School of Public Health. As his Master's thesis he formulated a plan for greater State support of public health, one that would strengthen local health work and foster a stronger relationship between the California State and the county departments of health. The plan entailed State appropriation of funds for county health departments. To be eligible, the local departments were required to meet standards set by a newly formed California Conference of Local Health Officers (CCLHO) in collaboration with the State Department of Public Health, which administered the program. Merrill and Halverson managed to put that arrangement into effect during the early 1950s as a major new element of California's public health work. It helped attract competent county health officers, encouraged greater State–local collaboration, and enhanced public health activities throughout the State. Merrill was thus largely responsible for building a strong State–local public health network in California. The county departments took responsibility for most public health services and the State Department served as technical resource and program developer. The CCLHO became an official advisor to the State Department of Public Health and has continued as an influential organization.

Warren and Halverson's arrangement for California's public health service functioned well for about 25 years through the governorships of Republican Goodwin Knight and Democrat Pat Brown and the public health directors they appointed: Halverson, Merrill, and me.

Beginning in 1967, however, Governor Ronald Reagan broke sharply with Warren's philosophy of government. Reagan appointed administrators who mainly followed his very conservative ideology in controlling the bureaucracy and carried out political, roll-back efforts rather than professionally determined, forward-looking social programs. They essentially tore down the governmental structure that Warren had built. For example, a 1975 California Auditor General's report noted that in the Department of Public Health, "Fifty-four positions in the Department require the incumbent to have a more specialized background either in terms of education, or work history, or both. However, 14 of the 54, or 26 percent, of the total positions in the Department of Health requiring a specialized program oriented background were filled by employees whose education, training and work had been limited to fiscal expertise" (Auditor General, State of California, 1975). Further, the report observed that "accountability has not increased with 46 percent of the 93 top administrators changing job assignments five or more times since 1970." Reagan thus thoroughly disrupted the health and other social programs in California's government that the Warren-Knight-Brown era had fostered.

Upon entering the California State Department of Public Health early in 1946, I was eager to start a new thrust in public health work, namely, chronic disease control (described in chapter 4). Although Halverson initially had little sympathy for that notion, he later came to support the idea. The fact that federal funds became available for cancer control during 1946 provided the needed resource for the Department to establish a Bureau of Chronic Diseases. Halverson and Robert Dyar, who headed the Division of Preventive Medical Services and my immediate superior, agreed with the latter title in response to my argument that, just as the federal government was making funds available for cancer control, it would soon support efforts for dealing with heart and other chronic diseases. Because the public health approach to these problems would be similar, it would be wise to consolidate chronic disease control into one unit from the start, comparable to the scope of work in the Bureau of Acute Communicable Diseases.

THE BUREAU OF CHRONIC DISEASES

Because the initial funds came specifically for cancer control, we devoted resources during the early years of the Bureau to that purpose. However, we began seeking funds for research and other activities directed toward heart disease, other specific chronic conditions, and chronic disease as a whole. As we had anticipated, Congress subsequently did appropriate funds for public health work on heart disease, which we used along with monies that became available for epidemiologic research on chronic diseases and other projects. Fortunately, we were able to attract excellent people for what became strong heart disease, cancer, and diabetes epidemiology components in the Bureau of Chronic Diseases. These groups joined in the national enthusiasm for ferreting out what was responsible for the increasing occurrence of these diseases, their consequent disability, premature mortality, and means of controlling them.

The National Institutes of Health (NIH) grew rapidly during the years following World War II, spearheaded by its expanding medical science constituency. We were extremely fortunate in the extent to which that agency's grants facilitated our Bureau's research work in those days despite the Institution's major emphasis on determining the mechanisms of disease and how to intervene in them.

In 1971 President Nixon's declaration of "War on Cancer" and the consequent spurt in National Cancer Institute (NCI) funding attracted further attention to cancer and invigorated the struggle against the chronic diseases as a whole. Unfortunately, the public health arm of that effort proved relatively weak. Even though the 1937 congressional action establishing the National Cancer Institute (NCI), specified that effort should be directed toward disease control as well as toward conducting and supporting laboratory and clinical investigations, the basic scientists and biologically oriented medical scientists in effect "captured" the NCI and the whole of the National Institutes of Health (NIH) and gradually steered it largely toward supporting their investigations. The NIH hence has focused largely on finding the "magic bullets" for treatment of disease and the basic sciences underlying such efforts. Over the years it has relatively neglected determining how we can apply what is already available in the armamentarium for dealing with current and future health. Public health approaches to disease have thus not benefited nearly as much as basic and clinical sciences from the vast investment in the NIH during the second half of the twentieth century. Although the agency has continued to support some work aimed at elucidating the totality of disease causation and how it can be controlled in the population, and our California programs benefited greatly thereby, the NIH has concentrated on the biological mechanisms of disease occurrence rather than on its external origins and what can be done about them.

Although the Centers for Disease Control and Prevention was established in 1946, it concentrated essentially all its early efforts on communicable disease control, and only in more recent years has it incorporated a relatively small amount of chronic disease control activity, considering the extent of that health problem in the United States compared with communicable disease. Hence, chronic disease control by the major federal health agencies has lagged.

At the mid-century point those of us devoted to chronic disease control in the public health sense recognized the severe limitations of our arsenal for attacking what we regarded as the new epidemics. We therefore devoted our efforts mainly to epidemiological studies of their prevalence and causation. We especially studied the conditions in which people lived and what they did in those conditions that might be responsible for the epidemics.

In addition to epidemiological investigations, however, we were constantly on the lookout for technologies that showed promise of reducing the chronic disease toll. For example, the Papanicolaou-Traut test (as the Pap smear was originally known) became available for public health application during the 1940s. We were unsuccessful in rapidly converting the test into a public health tool, due to opposition by pathologists and the reluctance of public health officials to undertake a medical care service (chapter 4).

The major voluntary health agencies such as the American Cancer Society, the American Heart Association, and the American Lung Association have flourished during the past several decades, sponsoring disease research and control programs with funds raised by public subscription. As they were such important elements of California's chronic disease program we maintained extensive contact with these organizations and their state and local affiliates, often conducting joint operations with them to provide public and professional education about what can and should be done for chronic disease control. We also collaborated with other organizations that reflected the growing interest in establishing and improving services for infirm, older people's health needs such as nursing home care. In the Bureau of Chronic Diseases, however, we focused mainly on developing means of prevention through epidemiological studies. Some of our early projects aimed at disease control, for example expanding use of the Pap smear, did not engender much enthusiasm in the medical profession.

THE DIVISION OF PREVENTIVE MEDICAL SERVICES

As the Chronic Diseases Bureau Chief from 1946 to 1960 I served on Dyar's staff along with those heading other bureaus in the Division of Preventive Medical Services that were concerned with Acute Communicable Diseases, Tuberculosis, Maternal and Child Health, Crippled Children Service, Occupational Health, Hospital Planning and Construction, and Hospital Licensure. All Division and Bureau chiefs gathered monthly with Halverson to review progress, problems, and issues. Our bi-monthly Division staff meetings brought together ten lively people with high morale discussing their exciting work and developing plans for new public health ventures.

In 1960 Dyar persuaded Merrill, who had succeeded Halverson as Director, to allow him to start a new Division of Research. By that time the Department was considerably engaged in research concerning many aspects of public health, and Dyar saw the need and opportunity to maintain excellence in that regard and to expand the effort. He had also developed an educational program in which medical students from across the country took a summer assignment to a specific Department project and attended Dyar's public health seminars. It was a highly successful enterprise, with dozens of medical students scattered throughout the Department each summer undertaking productive work and livening things up. The venture became so successful that in 1959 only 35 could be admitted out of more than 600 applicants from 68 medical schools. In that program we were engaging future physicians in public health research and professional education, while extending public health service in California. Having such students around and responding to their questions certainly helped to maintain the quality of departmental work.

When Merrill asked me to head the Division of Preventive Medical Services replacing Dyar, I happily accepted because my interests were expanding to embrace public health more fully, stimulated in part by participating in the American Public Health Association's activities. It was an easy transition for me because the new duties involved mainly taking the chair among Bureau chief colleagues with whom I had grown up professionally. No reorganization seemed necessary to me, though an outsider might have viewed the situation differently.

Taking the Division position meant moving into a higher echelon and thus being on the Director's immediate staff, along with assuming additional responsibilities such as budgetary and professional oversight for all the preventive medical bureaus. It was still possible for me to continue research activities, particularly in the Human Population Laboratory (described in chapter 6). Also, I was being invited to spend more time in national voluntary health association activities, especially in their etiological studies (e.g., serving on the American Cancer Society's National Committee on Research on Etiology, and the American Heart Association's Council of Epidemiology).

MEDICAL SERVICES FOR HEALTH

Medical care was becoming more important to public health because advances in it offered greater opportunities for restoring and maintaining health in the population as a whole. At that time three medical care issues attracted the attention of some of us in the public health community: effectiveness, efficiency, and equity. The increasing effectiveness of medical care (i.e., what good it could actually do for health) sprang from rapid progress in its technology. The issues of efficiency and equity in its operations arose directly from the fact that medical care was becoming so costly as to become a substantial political issue.

Increasing the efficiency of medical care as one approach to tackling the cost problem stirred many in the public health arena to advocate regionalization, that is, arranging medical services that would bring care in a rational manner to both larger and smaller communities based on the appropriate geographic arrangement of resources in relation to population need. That differed sharply from simply advancing institutional interests, which had been the main motivation in medical care planning previously. New, expensive technology would be located in a few carefully selected centers rather than being spread helter-skelter, a pattern that was already wastefully increasing cost to the entire community. Developing and distributing medical expertise in a rational fashion would presumably maximize its health impact. However, the idea of limiting individual freedom of action by regionalization so enraged California's medical and hospital leaders that they were commonly said to have influenced the University of California's decision to deny Edward Rogers, a professor in the School of Public Health at Berkeley, a promised higher academic post because he was an early advocate of regionalization.

Maintaining the regional aspect and related quality of the California State Crippled Children's Service (CCS), which the Department's Bureau chief sought as a vital element of the program, required a constant struggle. CCS administrators had long insisted upon purchasing medical services to diagnose and treat the often very difficult health problems of children only from hospitals and physicians especially selected for their competence (i.e., those meeting certain professionally approved standards). For example, as cardiac surgery for children was developing, CCS approved payment for that purpose to only a few centers that were scattered about the State in as many places of excellence as were genuinely needed to build and maintain proper use of the new technology. Several of the state's medical-political leaders consistently attacked that policy as undercutting the "freedom" of physicians to do whatever they thought they were individually capable of doing, and being paid for it with public funds. One physician member of the California Medical Association's Council led a battle extending over many years to allow any physician, appropriately qualified or not, to be reimbursed by CCS for any procedure he or she chose to carry out. The CCS staff, supported by relevant medical specialists, managed to prevail on that issue of quality. The CCS Bureau Chief's leadership and persistence exemplified what public health can and should do in the struggle for quality in medical services.

The 1957–58 California Health Survey, which was linked to the National Health Survey at that time, obtained information about medical care and morbidity in the population. Californians reported a total of 5.9 physician visits per person per year; but six percent of the people (ten percent of persons over 65 years of age) had not seen a physician within the past five years. Only one fourth of the state's residents over 65 years of age had any hospital insurance. Such data from California and many other sources facilitated passage of the Medicare Act in 1965.

Coinciding with my growing participation in national public health medical care developments, such as chairing the American Public Health Association Committee on Medical Care Administration, my duties as chief of the Preventive Medical Services Division included general supervision of all departmental medical care activities: traditional public health clinical services directed toward communicable disease control, the Hospital Planning and Construction program, and the Crippled Children's Service.

Funds made available by the federal Hill-Burton legislation and appropriations generated the Department's hospital construction program. Responding to the obvious need for additional hospital beds throughout the country, that legislation provided funds necessary to build hospitals according to a planned system of priorities established by each state for public and nonprofit facilities. The California program embraced regional planning for beds and related facilities to meet the hospital service needs of the State's expanding population, and then for selecting local, nonprofit or public agencies to which federal and state-matched funds would be allocated to cover two-thirds of the construction costs, with only one-third required from local government or voluntary sources. That program's leaders had established effective arrangements for fair allocations and reasonably smooth relationships with the relevant parties throughout the State involved in setting the priorities for distributing the available funds, and in dealing with stiff competition among regional hospital interests. As a statutory body the Hospital Advisory Council regularly reviewed and approved the staff work and recommendations. By the early 1960s we recognized that the Kaiser Health Plan and perhaps other influences that were curtailing hospital usage were reducing California's hospital need from the traditional 4.5 beds per 1,000 people to a substantially lower level. However, the vigorous demands from various regions of the State to use all available construction monies led to overbuilding California's hospital facilities from which, I regret, we have suffered for several years and have only recently been recovering.

When responsibility for administering the new Medicaid program came to the states, California was one of the first to seize the opportunity of obtaining federal funds to help pay for medical and related services for people below a certain income level, starting in March 1966. Some of us in the Department had participated in the legislative and implementation process both nationally and within California. (My wife favors a picture of me with President Johnson signing the Medicare-Medicaid legislation.) The administrator of the California Health and Welfare Agency asked us in the Department of Public Health to formulate the first year's Medicaid budget based on the available federal dollars; our proposed budget turned out to be very accurate in substantially meeting the need with the funds that had been appropriated. My role in initiating MediCal, as it was called in California, was to push for comprehensive care, rather than restricting the scope of service as several other states were doing; to advocate quality as had already been established in the Crippled Children's Service; and to help prepare the first budget. The extent of service and budget were, of course, intimately linked. Unfortunately, during Reagan's administration the budgeted amounts were not sufficient to cover comprehensive medical services, especially with poor cost controls.

Administrative responsibility for MediCal, however, went at the outset to the welfare agency, consistent with organized medicine's view and the prevailing political attitude that poor people's medical services—just like food, shelter, or any commodity for them—should be purchased in the welfare mode. The welfare agency would certify beneficiaries as eligible and the latter would then be free to select medical and related services on the open market just as they would buy groceries, except that the State would pay the vendors directly. That, of course, was quite different from the Crippled Children's Services or the subsequent California's Public Employee Retirement System (PERS) medical program, which seriously tried to safegaurd the quality of health services purchased with public funds by setting and implementing quality standards for the services. Subsequently, the Health and Welfare Agency established a new office for the MediCal program, the Office of Health Care Services (OHCS), which augmented those already in the Agency—Public Health, Social Welfare, Mental Hygiene, and Rehabilitation. The OHCS mainly contracted out the administrative services for payments to physicians, other practitioners, and hospitals and nursing homes, but it largely maintained the welfare mode of operation.

By November 1996, nearly half of California's licensed physicians were participating in the MediCal program only minimally or not at all. They were providing less than five percent of all MediCal physician services whereas about five percent of the participating physicians were providing 45 percent of the total MediCal services.

A member of our staff conducted a study of the quality of care in MediCal by investigating the extent of "shot-doctoring," which is providing injections of mainly useless substances to patients, whatever their health problems, and collecting the fee for the procedure. From the program's fee-for-service payment records we ascertained the names of physicians who, instead of the usual approximately 5–10 injections, gave as many as 50 and even more than 100 injections per 100 patients seen. Those submitting claims for such large numbers of injections per 100 patient visits obviously were practicing very poor medicine. The results indicated a need for action, but none was taken because the State Health and Welfare administrator feared that it would evoke hostility from organized medicine, which sought to protect physicians in almost whatever they did in their practices. Thus, the MediCal program immediately began attracting and even encouraging a brand of medicine contrary to that provided in CCS; essentially no attempt was made to deal with effectiveness or efficiency in the MediCal program. Welfare-type medical service administration went almost exclusively toward equity, called "access to the system," no matter how poor the services in the system were. Only in recent years have policy makers begun to consider ascertaining and improving the quality of medical services in public programs.

Besides the shot doctors, problem practitioners were also claiming payments for thousands of tonsillectomies that were performed as "preventive care," a procedure that even then was largely regarded by expert pediatricians as outmoded for such routine practice. Detailed examination of sample physicians' records indicated that many of them were providing services substantially below a reasonable quality. These cases were referred to the Office of Health Care Services, and I tried unsuccessfully to persuade the Health and Welfare agency head to look further into them for possible quality deficiencies and appropriate action. We recognized and emphasized that no provider should be judged or disciplined on the basis of the statistical record alone—although it does provide a basis for appropriate query about service quality—but the top State administrators declined taking any action for fear of alienating the medical profession.

During 1960, his first year in office and my first year as Division of Preventive Medical Services chief, Governor Brown charged me personally with a special assignment in the medical care field. He asked me to serve as staff director for the Governor's Committee on Medical Aid and Health (described in chapter 5). Brown also appointed me to the Board for California's Public Employment and Retirement Service (PERS) when that agency was first given statutory responsibility for a health benefits program (also described in chapter 5). As the only physician in the group, I was called upon to play a significant role.

ENVIRONMENTAL POLICIES AND ACTION FOR PUBLIC HEALTH

Environmental measures, such as for control of bacterial contamination of water and pasteurization of milk, had long been a feature of public health. The main advantages of such interventions were that, once in place, they required only maintenance, without repeated interventions. New aspects of the environment were attracting the attention of public health administrators, for example, in the mid 1950s when Los Angeles air pollution became more than a joke (described in chapter 5).

Also by the 1950s, far-sighted people were anticipating the time when Californians would have to reuse their water discharges for various purposes. Until that time the usual public health policy called for one standard for water that would be distributed to the public, namely, all of it must be drinkable (potable). Sanitarians traditionally had fought bitterly against allowing more than one standard for water, for fear of cross-connections in plumbing that would deliver polluted water to the public for drinking. Despite that concern Frank Stead, a public health engineer and Chief of Environmental Health in the Department, and some others foresaw the need for more water to be used in California than could be made potable by available technology. He strongly supported the Santee project in San Diego, which aimed at demonstrating that water that did not meet potable standards could be made useful for some purposes instead of being dumped to waste in sewage. Uses of Santee Lake, into which contaminated water flowed and was then partially treated and monitored, were gradually expanded to include boating and fishing in order to demonstrate that water from sewage, when properly treated and managed, could be reused safely. California is still grappling with the problem of scarce water for its expanding population and industry. As a prototype, the Santee project established one path for dealing with the problem. The difficulty has been complicated in recent years by having to deal not only with human discharges but also with contamination by toxic chemicals and, near the coast, with sea water. As of this writing, planning is underway in Orange County (between Los Angeles and San Diego Counties) to deposit treated domestic and other waste water into the ground water supply and thus save it, rather than discharging it into streams or the ocean.

Beyond special projects, such as Santee and developing air pollution standards, the Department's Division of Environmental Health has maintained surveillance over the traditional water, milk, and other systems for sanitary control and has provided technical assistance to those responsible for their maintenance. That is a highly important and substantial task.

INFLUENCES ON BEHAVIOR FOR PUBLIC HEALTH

In addition to environmental measures and medical services the third way to protect and advance health is through influencing behavior, for which the Department included a Bureau of Health Education. That unit, like its contemporary bureaus around the country at the mid-century point, had grown out of the public health tradition of urging people to adopt sanitary habits such as "Don't spit" and "Wash your hands," and to achieve personally healthful behavior with appeals to "Brush your teeth" and "See your doctor early in pregnancy." These slogans were used to support the campaigns directed toward safeguarding maternal health and combating communicable diseases during the first half of the twentieth century.

By the 1950s and 1960s, however, it became evident that a new set of health problems was upon us, the chronic diseases that resulted from what some people did in their everyday lives—eat too much, smoke cigarettes, fail to exercise, and drink alcoholic beverages excessively—just as what individual people did regarding their personal sanitation often contributed to health problems. Hence, public health began to emphasize what was known both about persuading individuals to adopt healthful behavior and about the circumstances inducing it. More sophisticated ways of trying to influence individual behavior in a healthful direction were only one component in the move toward better health through affecting what people did in their everyday lives. In addition and increasingly stressed, newer public health endeavors aimed at changing the actual situations in which people make decisions about their behavior, such as the price and availability of cigarettes, the places where one can smoke, and cigarette advertising; these were recognized as effective beyond appeals to individuals. Public health thus advanced in these directions toward controlling the many behaviors that were then being recognized as adversely affecting health.

Armed at first mainly with concepts derived primarily from individual psychology, for health educators that at first meant trying to persuade each person to live in ways that would not endanger his or her health. Although some efforts had been undertaken decades earlier to combat smoking and excessive drinking, these attempts had been largely colored with a moralistic approach. Now, scientific evidence concerning their health damage was becoming the rationale for such endeavors. The main thrust in health education, however, was still to persuade people as individuals at risk to adopt more healthful behaviors.

In dealing with unhealthful behavior public health, however, increasingly turned toward what a future Institute of Medicine report called the mission of public health, that is, to establish "the conditions in which people can be healthy" (Institute of Medicine, 1988). The focus became how to create circumstances that discourage people from smoking rather than trying to persuade them, one by one, to avoid the practice. Achieving healthful behavioral conditions was thus joined to medical service and environmental conditions. Bringing situations that affect behavior into this public health concept has often entailed conflict with those industrial forces whose products endanger health, but that seek to establish conditions that induce unhealthful behavior, such as unrestricted advertising of harmful products. Hence in the case of cigarettes we are beginning to recognize that what the tobacco industry does, not the smoker, is the target.

That same kind of understanding, fortunately, seems already to be affecting some segments of the food industry whose profits have depended on promoting food and drink consumption patterns that harm health. A few elements of the fast food industry are now introducing salads and other nutritious fare as an alternative to their current high fat, high sugar offerings. Public health leaders are also asking education authorities to abandon revenues from school sales of food and drink that are now injuring their students' health, and instead to provide healthful food and drink in the lunchroom and vending machines. Moving beyond persuasion, in some situations legislation is being adopted; for example, California has recently passed a law banning sodas from schools.

DEPARTMENTAL MISSION FOR THE 1960s

The 1961 California Department of Public Health annual report specified its mission to be "the achievement and maintenance of a safe and healthful environment [which we understood to mean the sociobehavioral as well as the physical environment] and an adequate program of medical care services for the entire population" in order to reach three objectives: "(1) the preservation and prolongation of life, (2) the prevention of disease and poisoning, and (3) the promotion of optimum health." The Department saw as its functions (1) to discharge the specific responsibilities assigned by law, (2) to bring about an efficient administration by local health departments of the general public health statutes and regulations, and (3) to maintain a program of investigation and research designed to provide continuing knowledge of the health status of the people of California, to identify conditions responsible for ill health, and to develop new technical and administrative methods of disease prevention and control. That statement guided the Department during the early 1960s when I served as Chief, Division of Preventive Medical Services, and continued through the 1965–1967 period when I was Director of the Department.

BECOMING DIRECTOR OF THE DEPARTMENT

In 1965, when Merrill accepted the medical directorship of the federal Agency for International Development in Washington, DC, then-Governor Pat Brown appointed me to succeed Merrill as State Director of Public Health. My two-and-a-half year tenure as Director mainly involved continuing what Halverson and Merrill had initiated during the preceding two decades. It was also the period when the Human Population Laboratory in Alameda County began operations (described in chapter 6).

I had known Governor Brown since about 1950 when he was serving as San Francisco District Attorney and we had some interaction concerning our mutual interest in controlling alcoholism. During his 1958 gubernatorial campaign, when he appeared at a Republican Women-for-Brown garden party in Berkeley, my 13-year-old son saw an announcement for the affair and, since I had mentioned knowing Brown, Steve asked me to take him to the event. As we were standing in the reception line, I wondered somewhat anxiously whether the nominee would recognize me and thus validate my account of knowing him. We had met only a few times and Brown, as a politician, had met thousands of people, so I anticipated having to introduce myself and my son. When we came up to Brown, however, he hailed me vigorously, "Hi, Doctor," and after I introduced my son, he pulled me over and exclaimed into my ear, "Glad to see you, but . . . what the hell are you doing here?"

Appointment as Director of Public Health entailed not only assuming responsibility for all departmental activities but also establishing and maintaining relationships with many other groups: various officials in the State administration, legislators and their staffs, voluntary health organizations, local health departments and other health agencies, and professional health societies. In that context some individuals stood out in my eyes, for example, a retired San Francisco merchant named Lawrence Arnstein. In devoting himself to several health endeavors, Arnstein had established effective channels to key people who knew and respected his knowledge, sage advice, and selflessness. He offered me bits of advice such as, "Call a meeting only with a clear purpose and when knowing what every attendant will say," and "You can accomplish anything in public health if you don't care who gets the credit." While perhaps not to be followed slavishly Arnstein's precepts were useful guides.

Brown's administration (1959–1966) dealt rather lightly with the State Department of Public Health. Paul Ward, then Secretary of the Health and Welfare Agency to whom as State Director of Public Health I reported administratively, left health matters almost entirely to the Department and the State Board of Health. During most of the 1960s, we were fortunate to have Roger Egberg as chair of the State Board of Health, after which he became Assistant Secretary for Health in the federal administration. Although Ward rejected some of my specific proposals as the Department's Director, he generally strongly supported our budget requests to carry out the wide scope of activities in which the Department was already engaged, and some new ventures. In those days the Board of Health had considerable authority, including the adoption of rules and regulations having the force of law and maintaining surveillance of public health in the state, particularly what the Department was doing about it. Subsequently, such responsibilities were taken back by Governor Reagan during his first term and the State Board of Health was shredded. These latter steps moved decisions about public health into the political machinery and away from the expertise that Warren had nurtured.

When I succeeded Merrill as Director, the Department consisted of the same major elements that most large states included in their health departments, though their structures varied somewhat. Having worked in the Department for almost 20 years and in effect having "grown up" professionally during its rapid expansion, I felt entirely comfortable in taking the leadership, especially with a strong connection to the State administration under Pat Brown.

SCOPE OF DEPARTMENTAL AND DIRECTOR'S ACTIVITIES

Among the Department's seven divisions Local Health Services (LHS), though relatively small in number of personnel, played a key departmental role by maintaining close liaison with the county and city health departments that covered essentially the entire state. The Division worked primarily through the California Conference of Local Health Officers (CCLHO) in building consensus for establishing standards for the local health departments and introducing new programs. Diplomacy was LHS's major tool, not only in guiding the local health officer community but also in helping resolve the inevitable tensions that would arise between local health officials and the people responsible for leading the programs in the other Divisions of the State Department of Public Health. Those state program chiefs typically had firm ideas about what should be done in their domains throughout the state, but when resistance was encountered in local jurisdictions where the health officer determined what would be done, LHS would help settle matters. The CCLHO had already functioned effectively for more than a decade as the core element linking

California state and local public health endeavor, and it continued to do so.

Dealing with Preventive Medical Services (PMS), having come directly from that Division into the Director's office, entailed my viewing it now in the context of the entire Department. The Division included the several bureaus concerned with traditional aspects of public health such as acute communicable disease control, tuberculosis, and maternal and child health, as well as some relatively new programs such as chronic disease and hospital planning and construction. The Bureau of Acute Communicable Diseases (ACD) included several epidemiologists who investigated outbreaks that extended over several counties, provided technical assistance to local health department epidemiologists and other personnel, and promoted and monitored acute communicable disease control measures, such as the extent of immunization against various diseases. Among the several elements in the Department, ACD was generally regarded by the public and its political leaders as providing the most crucial public health service.

Maternal and Child Health services (MCH), since the 1921 Sheppard-Towner Act first made federal funds available for the purpose, had also become ingrained in state and local public health endeavor. As in the case of acute communicable disease control, maternal and child health services had made tremendous strides during the first two-thirds of the twentieth century; but both the public and those devoted to the field professionally sought further advances and made it a popular program.

Beyond maintaining such traditional programs, however, about the middle of the twentieth century state public health departments began moving against other health problems, often with federal funds that were sometimes matched by state and local governments. Chronic disease was one such target, illustrated by the California experience (described in chapter 4).

The Crippled Children's Service, which was the Department's most direct medical care program, utilized State and federal funds earmarked for the purpose of identifying youngsters with congenital and other severe impairments, and then arranging for appropriate medical, hospital, and related services. Although an essentially nationwide public health activity, the California CCS program had become relatively extensive. Though it was initiated mainly as an orthopedic service, Marcia Hays, as the program's director, had worked effectively with community groups to expand it greatly; many medical and surgical conditions qualified for support. Dr. Hays insisted on high standards for the care that the funds would provide in selected private, nonprofit, and county Hospitals. The programs thus helped stimulate excellent children's hospital services generally in the State.

Another highly significant departmental activity was carrying out the Bureau of Hospitals' responsibility for licensure of hospitals and nursing homes as well as for hospital planning and construction. By the time I came into the Director's position Gordon Cumming had already built that Bureau into a large-scale operation with extensive connections to California's hospital and medical communities. Hospital licensure was conducted with an inspection staff whose members made periodic visits to hospitals and nursing homes to ensure their compliance with State Board of Health standards. Rarely was it necessary to suspend a licensee; alerting the operators to deficiencies usually sufficed to achieve correction; the Bureau's reputation for toughness encouraged prompt action.

What a state health director can do regarding medical services was exemplified in the 1965 event in South Los Angeles (Watts) which brought to light a severe blot on the California health scene. Poverty and other disadvantages that prevailed among the African-American people living there had provoked a riotous demonstration with burning, pillaging, and deaths. The report of a Commission headed by John McCone reviewed the background and recommended, among other things, improved hospital services in the area. Digging into the Watts situation we found that the Department's hospital planning had unintentionally, but actually, gerrymandered the South Los Angeles County area into four quarters. Each segment was combined with an area outside Watts that included hospital service adequate for the people living in those areas adjacent to Watts, but not really available to people living in Watts. This arrangement effectively denied federal–state hospital construction aid to a very needy area because the hospital areas into which Watts had been cordoned off did not really serve the people of Watts who were mainly poor and black and could not obtain hospital care at the "available" hospitals. A Watts resident reportedly had to be "$10 sick" to get hospital care, ten dollars being the taxi fare to the Los Angeles County General Hospital, the only place where such a person could then obtain inpatient care; a person sick enough for hospital admission could not handle the three bus transfers to get there and so had to have taxi fare. Upon reading the McCone Commission Report, by that time as State Health Director, I asked the Department's hospital planning staff for Watts' priority standing for Hill-Burton hospital construction funds. The rectangular area in South Los Angeles called Watts, where the social eruption had occurred, was neatly mapped off into the four adjacent hospital planning areas that did have adequate hospital facilities for their populations and thus were low on the priority list. The problem was that the Watts residents could not gain admission to these closer, private facilities and therefore were forced to obtain hospital services only in the County facility.

I proposed solving the matter very simply: "Just give me a pencil." I then drew on the map a rectangle embracing the relevant area and projected it as a new Hospital Plan Service Area. Having no hospital facilities, the new Watts area thus immediately went to the top of the federal–state funding priority list. Of course, the situation had to be handled officially through the planning bodies, but the upshot was that Los Angeles County was able to appropriate the one-third County match for the Hill-Burton funds and thereby build the King Hospital. Subsequently, the UCLA and USC Medical Schools' support enabled it to become the King/Drew Medical Center.

Medical Services

By the 1960s medical care had become so obviously significant for health that providing medical services for all people was gaining considerable prominence on the national political scene. In 1965 Congress enacted the Medicare-Medicaid legislation that inaugurated the nation's greatest medical service advancement during the latter half of the century. It finally linked medical care to Social Security as Franklin Roosevelt had desired in 1935 but had judged not then feasible politically; it also created a federal–state program providing medical services to certain welfare recipients. The legislation aroused considerable excitement among public health-medical care advocates. Many of us journeyed to Washington to support it and suggest amendments. In testifying before a Congressional committee, for example, I proposed that payments for nursing home care should be limited to institutions where the service was overseen by the medical staff of a nearby hospital with which the nursing home would thereby be connected. Although physician-staffed committees in the hospitals were by no means fully assuring good care for hospitalized patients, they were making reasonable progress in that direction. Extending organized physician oversight to nursing home care seemed a good way of improving services to patients admitted to such institutions. Otherwise the (mainly proprietary) nursing homes would largely suck up the increased federal–state funds while providing the same inadequate and often harmful care that prevailed at the time. Public welfare protagonists had long sought funds for medical services in the same mode as for food and shelter, not realizing that in the case of professional health care services it was important to seek and achieve quality standards. Physician organizations as well as conservatives generally joined public welfare workers in asserting "just allocate some money." Differences on the issue between Wilbur Cohen, a professional social worker and Johnson administrator, and me were so sharp that Phil Lee, Assistant Secretary for Health, who was seated between us during congressional testimony, literally stretched out his long arms over our chests to restrain the two colleagues at his right and left sides. Cohen, having far greater political insight and effectiveness than I did, prevailed, but the recurring nursing home scandals sadden me greatly. Nursing home patients still deserve far better care than they generally receive.

Environmental Health Services

The Division of Environmental Health carried responsibility for protecting people from hazards of contaminated water and food and polluted air. To a considerable extent appropriate measures had long been established (e.g., sewage disposal, water treatment, and pasteurization of milk). Even though routinely operating such safeguards had become the province of other agencies, constant public health vigilance was necessary, particularly in view of the growth of California's population. Also, concern about new threats strongly motivated the Division's public health engineers, exemplified by their participation in setting standards for air pollution. Potential harm from exposure to radiation, chemicals, and microorganisms was also arousing popular concern. Seeking to differentiate the imagined from the real hazards, ascertaining the latter's origin and nature of environmental spread, and then to developing standards for effective control measures posed significant problems for the Department's Division of Environment Health. That role has increasingly been adopted by state environmental health agencies in general, but responsibility for actually operating the control measures, once established, has usually passed to other hands. Of all elements in the California Department of Public Health, Environmental Health made me feel the most dependent because of the staff's great technical competence in matters that I least understood. Staff capability in all parts of the Department exceeded mine, but at least I had a better understanding of what some were doing than I did in the case of environmental health.

Bureau of Occupational Health personnel investigated work conditions that gave rise to disease and disability. The Bureau did not rest on what had already been discovered about occupational factors in disease, but vigorously pursued other situations in which there was reason to suspect adverse health consequences from work. The Bureau Chief became a national leader in the investigation of asbestos as a cause of severe pulmonary disease, which often resulted in death, and in the subsequent battles to control exposure and compensate the victims.

The 1960s presented some bizarre situations for public health environmental decisions, precipitated by the new "styles" of that decade. One Friday afternoon about 4:45 P.M. we received a telephone call informing us that a substantial amount of LSD, the psychotropic drug, had been dumped into the Marin County water tank (just north across the Bay from San Francisco), a holding tank for water that was then distributed directly to residences. We immediately undertook an investigation of the local situation which disclosed no evidence that anyone had broken into the secured area. No quick laboratory test for LSD in such a situation was available. A conference in my office involving engineers, laboratory, and public information personnel resulted in a decision to run the water to waste and simultaneously refill the reservoir with fresh water, without public announcement. In retrospect, the incident could have generated considerable excitement, though there was no real evidence of chemical pollution. One young staff engineer remarked about the potential effect of LSD in the water supply, "In Marin County (with its population of middle-class Yuppies) what difference would it make anyway!"

Laboratory Services

Beginning with the bacteriological era in the late nineteenth century public health agencies had developed and relied on Public Health Laboratory services to guide communicable disease control efforts. They provided the routine scientific underpinning for such major public health activities. At first these services were used to identify bacterial agents responsible for epidemics, and then to help diagnose disease in individual patients in order to facilitate appropriate treatment. As science advanced, new procedures were incorporated into the public health laboratory armamentarium, including those for detecting viral and chemical agents that may damage health. In addition to providing community service, health department laboratories often carried out research jointly with university laboratories. The California State Department of Public Health Division of Laboratories served as an effective and constantly advancing enterprise that supported the Department's communicable disease control and environmental health work. It also served as a reference laboratory for local health department laboratories and for clinical facilities around the State. That meant checking specimens as requested and participating in studies of complex situations. Improving and maintaining laboratory service throughout California was an important Department aim.

Another major support element on which the Department relied heavily was the Division of Administration, which contained bureaus responsible for fiscal and personnel matters throughout the Department. In addition the fundamental public health role in maintaining vital statistics (birth, death, and communicable disease) based on reports from local health departments was housed in the Division's Bureau of Vital Statistics. A somewhat unusual feature in the California State Department of Health was inclusion of the Bureau of Health Education in the Division of Administration. Although that Bureau's leader sometimes fretted at being linked to the Division of Administration, placement there may have reflected the relative weakness at the time of what health education was regarded as capable of accomplishing. It surely didn't belong in either of the two largest program Divisions, Preventive Medical Services or Environmental Health. Public health espoused the importance of an informed public, but the significance of behavior in the current epidemic diseases such as cardiovascular disease and cancer had only recently been recognized; evidence for effectiveness of measures to influence health-related behavior was yet to develop. The Surgeon General's Report on Smoking and Health had just been published in 1964. Lack of knowledge about behavior and health in part motivated our development of the Human Population Laboratory in Alameda County.

Initiating the Department's Division of Research during the early 1960s has already been noted earlier in this chapter. Dyar's considerable epidemiological expertise greatly strengthened the Department's research enterprise, and he reveled in the greater time he could devote to the medical student program he had developed. The fact that in 1965 as Director I was above Dyar in the hierarchy occasioned no difficulty, although he had brought me as a young medical officer into the Division of Preventive Medical Services that he then headed. The working situation was so comfortable that I don't recall ever thinking about that fact until writing this paragraph. It induces me again to reflect on the excellent ambience that Halverson and Merrill had established in the Department.

Finally, the newest unit in those days, the Division of Alcoholism, was created because that condition was evoking substantial public interest and political expectation of what public health could do about it. The Department's action reflected growing recognition that the condition is fundamentally a health problem rather than simply an occasional and relatively minor matter for the police. Failure of the Bureau of Chronic Diseases to undertake activities in that health area may also have heightened the passion with which advocates for alcoholism control advanced their demand for a separate, major place on the state's public health agenda.

A TOUR AS PRESIDENT OF THE AMERICAN PUBLIC HEALTH ASSOCIATION

Having served the American Public Health Association in various capacities including Governing Council membership, I was elected President of the Association for 1969. Besides engaging in the typical activities in such a post, I undertook with Paul Cornely, the President-elect, a tour of the United States, to examine firsthand common environmental and medical care situations giving rise to health problems. "We believed it was time for health professionals to see, hear, and smell these situations which characterize the lives of millions of Americans, rather than to limit our view of the problems to health statistics, patients in clinics and laboratory specimens" (American Public Health Association, 1970, p. IV).

The journey took us to a Mexican-American barrio in Houston, rural Tulare County in California, juvenile and adult prisons in Atlanta, the Potomac River in Washington, D.C., homes of off-reservation Indians in Great Falls, Montana, and the south side of Chicago. We found "circumstances that can only be called health brutality . . . (that) . . . seem designed to break the human spirit" (American Public Health Association, 1970, p. IV).

Though we published our findings and journalists and some local officials accompanied us, the tour received practically no national press attention.

DEPARTURE FROM THE DEPARTMENT

After defeating Brown for re-election, Reagan took office rather ostentatiously at 12:01 A.M., January 1, 1967. My appointment extended through December 31, 1967, since Warren and Halverson had arranged statutorily for the Public Health Director to serve a four-year term extending through the first year of a new Governor's term. They reasoned that the Director of Public Health should be an expert, professional, non-political appointee and that an incoming Governor and the incumbent Public Health Director would come to be satisfied with each other. The idea worked well for 25 years, but that tradition in California public health work that reflected the Warren-initiated excellence in State government was broken by Ronald Reagan when he became governor in 1967. It is not just that he opposed "bureaucracy" and "high taxes"; he simply did not believe in government maintaining responsibility for welfare, education, public health, or its many other generally accepted functions. He would make all these matters for private enterprise. (Arriving on the national scene, he even tried to turn national defense over to the private sector and the generals, thus seriously violating Eisenhower's warning about the military-industrial complex.)

My experience with Reagan lasted one year into his first term. Shortly after his inauguration a member of his staff visited me to convey the Governor's wish that I resign as Director of Public Health so that he could put his "whole new team" in place, although my term was supposed to last through 1967. The notion that a new governor and the public health director would get used to one another had prevailed for almost a quarter-century. Actually, I was no more eager to work for Reagan than he wanted me in his administration, but believing that the tradition supported public health I asked for and was given the opportunity to consult colleagues in the public health, medicine, and hospital worlds. Though some had vigorously opposed some of my policies and told me they had voted for Reagan, they unanimously insisted that I should stay. They all seemed proud of the Department, wanted it preserved, and did not want the statutory arrangement disrupted. Acting on that advice I refused to resign. After some further buffeting, Spencer Williams, in Reagan's Health and Welfare cabinet post, finally told me that I could stay for the final year of my term without any further harassment. Toward the year's end, however, it became clear that Reagan would not reappoint me for another four-year term. Instead his staff proposed that I continue on a day-to-day basis. That, of course, was completely unsatisfactory to me, and I had already almost completed negotiations to become a UCLA Professor of Public Health.

Meanwhile Spencer Williams was publicly proclaiming my excellence as a public health officer and recommending my reappointment. Reagan, however, decided against that action. When newspaper reporters asked him why he was "firing" the Director of Public Health, who was then President of the American Public Health Association, Governor Reagan responded that, while I was technically competent, we had a difference in philosophy. When asked for comment on the latter point, I answered that although the Governor and I had encountered some differences, on that point we were thoroughly agreed.

Actually, several public health professionals left the Department when California entered the Reagan era to accept professorships in the University of California system; at the Universities of Michigan, Arizona, and Washington; and at Harvard, Yale, and USC, where their outstanding qualifications and productivity were well recognized.

Believing that the State Board of Health had long constituted a major Departmental bulwark against imposition of a Governor's beliefs about public health, a Reagan-appointed task force attacked the Board in a closely held but leaked report that was not given to the Board itself. Reacting to that report and other Reagan administration health-related actions, Roger Egeberg, then President of the Board as well as Dean of the University of Southern California Medical School, was quoted in a newspaper as vigorously opposing the efforts to "scuttle" the Department and shouting, "I am goddamned mad and I do not propose to be quoted as saying I am very angry."

Major memories of my participation in California's public health administration were thus the continuity of public health leadership and programming established by Earl Warren as Governor and extending through Goodwin Knight's and Pat Brown's terms, development of chronic disease control, the Human Population Laboratory in Alameda County, air pollution control, the strong relationship that evolved between the State Department of Health and local health departments, implementation of the MediCal program, actions aimed at improving the quality of medical services for Californians, and termination of my service by Ronald Reagan as Governor.

Experience as a Departmental administrator confirmed and extended for me the larger view of public health described in chapter 5 (see Table 4, p. 71). I came to realize that epidemiology and associated biostatistics constitute the essential public health arm for diagnosing the nature, extent, and causation of community health problems. Treatment embraces three important elements: (1) medical (and related) services, both preventive and therapeutic, (2) environmental health services, which include the great advantage of not requiring individual action after public consensus is reached and appropriate social action taken, and (3) influencing behavior, especially by achieving conditions that favor healthful daily habit patterns regarding exercise, use of alcohol and tobacco, and personal hygiene. Although my experience as described in this account may seem to emphasize medical services, I want to stress my belief that, though vitally important, they do not affect health as much as behavior does. Environmental health services, originally the basic element of public health, continue to play a key role today when our technological manipulation of the physical and chemical conditions of our lives has become so great.

All three kinds of public health services must be included in a comprehensive advance toward health and embraced in public health administration.

International Health

9

From the public health perspective international health means the health status around the world, the factors that determine it, and the means of dealing with it. The trend toward a global economy with its technical advances is creating one world and vastly affecting its health problems. Continuing interdependence among countries with respect to health is strikingly illustrated by the world-wide epidemic of Severe Acute Respiratory Syndrome (SARS) as this is being written. Protection of international health is thus attracting renewed attention.

A fundamental feature of the current international situation is the well-known division of nations into the so-called developed and developing world, the former being the highly industrialized and more affluent countries, and the latter, those where primitive economies and overwhelming poverty prevail. The huge and increasing gap results from extending into the twenty-first century the imperial powers' domination and exploitation of the less advantaged nations during the nineteenth and twentieth centuries. That phenomenon has continued through the twentieth century. Examples include the (recently curtailed) marketing of powdered milk as the "modern" alternative to breast feeding, even when the necessity of mixing it with local polluted water obviously caused tremendous mortality from infant diarrheal disease, and breast feeding is advocated as a health measure in those nations that exported the powdered milk; and the continued marketing of cigarettes to peoples of the developing world, which is supported by the "advanced" nations, even though the huge adverse impact on health is well known and being controlled in the developed countries by sales restrictions. These trends exemplify what may properly be called the "new colonialism."

171

Even efforts by some activists in the developed countries to aid the less fortunate peoples have yielded negative results, for example, exporting "cancer control" to developing nations by cultivating high-tech tertiary care for cancer patients when the possible benefit is clearly limited to a small segment of the local population who can afford the care, while neglecting opportunities to advance against cancer among larger segments of the population that would be possible with less expenditure, for example, against cervical cancer. Such distortion of health expenditures is a major international health issue.

Large-scale war involving introduction of weapons causing mass destruction is a third phenomenon that severely affected health during the twentieth century. War has always yielded casualties, but development and use of weapons of mass destruction have increased its horror. World War I brought mustard gas to the front line and opened the path to development of other toxic and then biologic agents. Invention and stockpiling of the atom bomb has profoundly increased the potential for destruction. The nuclear bomb threat exists not only among nations but also within rogue bands of civilians who might obtain the weapon.

Global warming is still another international health problem confronting humanity as we enter the twenty-first century. As much media and scientific attention has focused on its consequences for biodiversity, substantial human health effects are also looming large. The steady melting of the polar ice packs and consequent raising of the sea level results in greater movement of salt into coastal rivers, thus denying people drinking water. Moreover, global warming is extending the range of disease-bearing insects, such as the anopheles mosquito that carries malaria, and disrupting some agricultural production. Although various bodies have adapted policy statements on the matter, little to counter the massive trend has actually been accomplished.

Population growth in many parts of the world is creating a huge set of health problems. That growth reflects multiple social forces: religious doctrines opposing birth control measures, producing more children to sustain family economy, and longer survival of people. It has already yielded considerable communicable disease and famine, and the trend toward overpopulation is still mainly uncontrolled.

Although public health has recently begun to grapple with some of these new challenges, global health efforts actually began long ago to prevent the international spread of communicable diseases when commerce between nations expanded. These efforts first took the form of quarantining vessels coming from distant lands and convening the International Health Conference in Paris in 1851. Not much was accomplished, however, until the beginning of the twentieth century with the development of the International Health Organization and the Pan American Sanitary Conference. These organizations fostered the exchange of information about the occurrence of major epidemic diseases and the adoption of sanitary conventions and quarantine regulations. Faced with huge health as well as economic and social problems following World War II, government leaders organized the United Nations Relief and Rehabilitation Administration (UNRRA), and then the World Health Organization (WHO). The latter was formed in 1948 as a specialized body of the United Nations for the purpose of furnishing practical assistance to various national health efforts and promoting international collaboration among health experts. The preamble to the WHO constitution asserts that "governments have a responsibility for the health of their peoples which can be fulfilled only by the provision of adequate health and social measures" (WHO, 1948). Subsequently, several developed nations adopted measures and formed agencies to advance health in less affluent countries: for example, the U.S. Agency for International Development (USAID).

For decades philanthropic foundations have undertaken international health programs, notably the Rockefeller, Ford, and Kellogg Foundations in the United States, and similar bodies in other countries. Numerous smaller organizations have entered the field, including church groups and recently "Doctors Without Borders." These non-governmental organizations (NGOs) have contributed substantially to international health work both in their direct activities and in pointing the way for governments to help meet the needs.

Meanwhile the World Health Organization has flourished. It established a headquarters office in Geneva, Switzerland, and six regional offices throughout the world that recruit experts from various countries to consult on WHO activities and to participate in its projects. In 1978 the WHO joined with the United Nations International Children's Emergency Fund (UNICEF) in the Alma Alta Declaration, asserting health to be a "fundamental human right," that "primary health care . . . constitutes the first element of a continuing health care process," and proposed "health for all by the year 2000" (World Health Organization and UNICEF, 1978).

The greatest international health achievement has, no doubt, been the eradication of smallpox, which had decimated untold numbers of people throughout the world over the centuries. That example has raised the prospect of similarly effective action against poliomyelitis, which already no longer occurs in North and South America and other major portions of the world; measles may be next on the agenda for extinction. Another significant step came with adoption of the infant mortality index

as a general measure of health. That has enabled analysts to compare
the health of various countries and to monitor progress in health improvement around the world, as well as in regions and segments of the populations within countries. More recently the WHO, particularly its European
office in Copenhagen, has been turning attention to the noncommunicable diseases. The International Agency for Cancer Research in Lyon,
France, has provided notable leadership in combating malignant neoplasms that have become such a major health problem throughout most
of the world.

THE INTERNATIONAL EPIDEMIOLOGICAL ASSOCIATION

The challenging precepts that the WHO put forward and the advances
nurtured by other agencies stimulated a global perspective among several
young physicians during the years following World War II. They realized
the immensity of the problems: extreme poverty and ignorance; gross
malnutrition; continuing tuberculosis, malaria, and other communicable
diseases; a scarcity of even ill-prepared health personnel; and the noncommunicable disease problems that were affecting people in the developed
countries and likely to spread to the whole world. Post-World War II
enthusiasm for applying medicine and epidemiology as tools for dealing
with health issues encouraged these young physicians to tackle such
difficult problems. They sensed that the generally favorable social climate
would support their efforts toward building international collaboration
in health work.

Two of those young physicians, John Pemberton in England and Harold Willard in the United States, who were seeking a scientific approach
to population health (epidemiology), and social factors in health and
disease control (social medicine), believed that exchanging information
on these topics among investigators in various countries would advance
the cause. With advice from the Scottish senior bacteriologist-epidemiolo-
gist, Robert Cruikshank, they formed the International Corresponding
Club (ICC) in Social Medicine to facilitate communication between physicians working for the most part in university departments of preventive
and social medicine throughout the world.

Growing out of our association in the ICC, several of us American
physicians who were pursuing social medicine and chronic disease epidemiology admired the ideas and achievements of our British epidemiology
colleagues. Jeremy Morris had shown that London bus conductors experienced lower coronary heart disease rates than drivers on the same buses,
and he attributed the discrepancy to a protective effect of physical exer-

tion on the job (Morris & Crawford, 1958). Richard Doll was carrying out his highly influential study demonstrating tobacco's adverse health effect among physicians (Doll & Hill, 1952). Archibald Cochrane developed the notion of clinical trials, first studying the outcomes of coronary heart disease patients whom he randomly assigned to either hospital or home treatment (Cochrane, 1972). Cochrane exemplified the group's ideological inclinations on both sides of the Atlantic: skepticism about the health value of many common medical procedures; eagerness to test all medical procedures scientifically; approaching health comprehensively through epidemiology; and politically, a profound anti-Fascism (Archie had fought on the Republican-Loyalist side against the Fascist Franco in the Spanish Civil War during the late 1930s). His initiative in applying epidemiology to determine the effectiveness of medical procedures was an early thrust toward what is now called "evidence-based medicine." The activity, which he initiated and now termed the Cochrane Collaboration, expresses his work's importance in improving medical care decision making. The Collaborative's service "preparing, maintaining, and promoting the accessibility of systematic reviews of the effects of health care interventions" is appealing to more and more physicians throughout the world (Bosch, 2003).

ICC members, supported by the Rockefeller Foundation, conducted their First International Scientific Meeting in 1957 in Noordwijk, the Netherlands, where the fifty-eight participants from twenty countries formed the International Epidemiological Association (IEA), with Robert Cruikshank as founding President. The Noordwijk meeting provided a marvelous opportunity for me to meet leading epidemiologists from several countries and learn about their work. Robert Cruikshank vigorously espoused "spreading the gospel" of epidemiology, thus combining in a phrase his Scottish theological and scientific background. His leadership inspired the attending epidemiologists from twenty countries to form the new organization with enthusiasm. The high quality of the papers at that first meeting engendered great pleasure, and joining colleagues with whom we were delighted to be associated gratified us all.

Determined to make the Association truly international, the IEA leadership scheduled the second meeting in Cali, Colombia. One of that 1959 session's attractive personalities was the socially minded local medical school Dean, Gabriel Velasquez. When asked the school's purpose, he responded, "To improve medical care for the people living in this beautiful valley." Medical education would probably be considerably enhanced if deans of medical schools elsewhere emphasized the same intent for people in their surrounding communities.

Thereafter, some Americans became more prominent in International Epidemiological Association affairs, particularly Kerr White, an epidemi-

ologist based at the University of North Carolina, who successfully sought
PL 480 funds to support Association meetings. Reflecting the UNRRA
and UN spirit following World War II, the U.S. Congress had appropriated
these PL 480 monies to encourage scientific and cultural exchange between the U.S. and certain other countries, including Yugoslavia. The
funds permitted the IEA to hold three meetings there in the 1960s and
early 1970s.

Having been elected to the Executive Council at Noordwijk and then
chairman of the IEA Council at the 1964 meeting, I presided at the 1968
Primosten, Yugoslavia, session. My principal goal as IEA president was
to spread the membership more vigorously into Eastern Europe, hoping
among other things to help mitigate the Cold War's adverse effects on
health science interchange. The fourteen countries represented at the
1968 meeting included Czechoslovakia, Poland, the USSR, and Yugoslavia, along with western European, North and South American, Asian,
and Middle Eastern nations.

A few days before the meeting in Primosten, the Soviets had invaded
and overpowered Czechoslovakia, in order to suppress the deviant ideas
that were emerging there. That action shocked our members, who were
devoted to peaceful internationalism and wanted the nations of the world
to engage in cultural exchange and scientific collaboration, not armed
conflict. The heavy-handed move cast a pall over the meeting. Two young
Czech epidemiologists came with their families intending to leave their
country, and at least one did find a position elsewhere, aided by a fellow
IEA member.

Thereafter, triennial sessions of the IEA in locations throughout the
world attracted growing participation by the increasing numbers of epidemiologists involved and the number of countries represented: in 1964,
there were 144 members from thirty countries, and in 1984, 1,371 members from ninety-eight countries. The leadership has included, for example, A. O. Lucas, a Nigerian who presided at the 1974 meeting in Brighton,
England; and J. Kostzewski, then the Minister of Health in Poland, who
served as president during 1977–81. By 1990 the IEA had become a
flourishing organization with almost 2,000 members. Seven hundred
from more than 60 countries attended the international meeting that
year in Los Angeles, where my wife, Devra, assisted Roger Detels, UCLA
School of Public Health Professor of Epidemiology and then IEA president, in organizing that congress. It has been my good fortune to attend
every one of the fourteen IEA international meetings, hosted in the
Netherlands, Colombia, Yugoslavia, England, Scotland, Canada, Finland,
the United States, Australia, Japan, and Italy. Viewing my bureau-top
photograph of those attending the original 1957 Noordwijk meeting still

gives me great pleasure. The leadership of the organization also indicates the IEA success in "spreading the gospel" of epidemiology; recent Executive Committee members have included epidemiologists from South Africa, Thailand, Chile, Saudi Arabia and India, as well as the United Kingdom, Germany, Japan, the U.S., and France.

As an important feature of IEA work, the *Journal of the International Epidemiology Association* has for decades published reports of epidemiological work from all parts of the globe. The IEA has also conducted several dozen regional meetings, each attracting hundreds of epidemiologists from the host and surrounding countries. I attended early ones, in Jamaica with Cruikshank in 1968, and in Ibadan, Nigeria, when the 1970 Biafran war ended. The IEA Council, in cooperation with local members, has organized sessions in Nairobi, Kenya; Baghdad, Iraq; Pattaya, Thailand; Bali, Indonesia; Victoria Falls, Zimbabwe; Salvador, Brazil; and other places throughout the world. The IEA has thus become a genuinely international society and has been highly successful in promoting epidemiology as a world-wide venture.

Associating with IEA colleagues and taking part in the growth of epidemiology internationally has given me great professional joy. I regard it a tremendous honor having been elected in 1984 to the first group of honorary IEA members, along with Richard Doll, the outstanding English epidemiologist; Carlos Gonzalez, a leading epidemiologist in Venezuela and member of the IEA Council; and Leo Kaprio, the distinguished Director of the WHO European office in Copenhagen. Especially exhilarating to contemplate, the many contributions of epidemiology to world health advances during the latter half of the twentieth century have taken magnificent form. They include smallpox eradication, the current and increasing potential for dealing similarly with both measles and poliomyelitis, the extensive control of thyroid disease with iodine, preventing eye disease with vitamin A, and the scientific bases for past and future progress against heart disease, cancer, and other chronic diseases.

OFFSHOOTS FROM NOORDWIJK

On the journey with me to Noordwijk for the founding meeting of the IEA, my son, Norman, insisted on placing Zermatt, Switzerland, on our itinerary. En route there from Paris, he explained his intent to climb the famous mountain, the Matterhorn. That struck me as a highly dangerous venture and aroused my alarm, but he was adamant. He asserted that he was well acquainted with what a Matterhorn ascent involved, and was thoroughly competent to carry it out. Emphasizing that we could spend only three nights and two days in Zermatt, I specified three conditions for his proposed climb. The first was that the weather had to be perfect, not just "all right." Second, his guide would have to satisfy me, and that would not be easy. Third, the test on which he indicated the guide would take him prior to starting the climb must show that Norman was an excellent climber, not just passable. Eager for the adventure, Norman accepted those conditions. I was confident that it would be impossible within the time available to satisfy all three of them.

We checked into the Zermatt Hotel after a late afternoon arrival. Soon he asked me to come downstairs to meet his new friend, a guide whom he had encountered in the boot shop. Norm introduced me to a young man who appeared to be the picture of health. His grandfather and father had been guides; and the young man himself had taken many people on the Matterhorn climb, he said, without any mishap. "Well," I thought, "that was only one condition." The next morning when they returned from the "test," the guide proposed that the two take a more difficult route up the Matterhorn than usual because Norman was such an excellent climber. The sun was shining brightly with no breeze and without a cloud in the sky. Undone by my handling of the difficult situation with the three conditions, I had to give consent, but I insisted that they follow the climb's regular course.

The two left that afternoon about 3:00 P.M. After camping overnight, an early start the next day would bring them to the mountain's top, and then back about noontime. As they departed I asked Norm to call me when he reached a telephone, about an hour out from the restaurant where I would be waiting the next noon. Walking back to the hotel I passed a cemetery where I paused to observe the ages at which people buried there had died. The stones gave devastating information: so-and-so from Nottingham died on the Matterhorn at the age of 17; the next, age 19 and also from England, had died on the Matterhorn; and so on. I spent the evening drinking with two psychiatrists from Yale, also guests at the hotel, who helped me considerably. The next morning about 10:00 A.M., I arrived at the restaurant where Norm and his guide would be returning, hoping that possibly they would reach the telephone earlier than expected. At 1:00 and then almost 2:00 P.M. with no call and all other parties that day having returned, I became frantic. Finally a few minutes after 2:00, Norman and his guide walked up to the restaurant. I ran out to greet him, never so happy and so angry at the same moment in my entire life. His explanation for not having made the telephone call was that when he arrived at the place, he found it would cost a franc and he felt it was not worth the expense. But then I was probably to blame for having indoctrinated him with such frugality.

Subsequent to the Noordwijk meeting, Karel Raska, Professor and Director of the Czechoslovakia Institute of Hygiene, invited me and a few other Western epidemiologists to participate in an Eastern European epidemiology meeting that he was hosting. Attendants came mainly from the U.S.S.R. and Czechoslovakia, with a few from other East European countries. Raska invited me to give the opening lecture in which I presented an epidemiological idea then spreading in the West and recounted earlier here, namely, that coronary heart disease, lung cancer, and the other major, current chronic disease epidemics resulted mainly from certain behaviors. These were associated with newly acquired affluence, especially too little physical demand on people, excessive caloric intake, cigarette smoking, and too much fat in the diet. I predicted that the chronic disease epidemics that were then severely affecting the Western European and North American regions would be spreading into Eastern Europe as more people there acquired better economic circumstances and adopted the causative behaviors, unless they were alerted and avoided the habits. Unfortunately, my prediction came true.

The leading Russian epidemiologist at the session immediately challenged that notion and me in particular. Speaking in excellent English (much to my discomfiture because my English presentation had to be translated into Russian, which most attendees understood), he called the idea that I had advocated utter nonsense. He asserted it to be an alien intrusion into an epidemiological meeting where everybody knew, he insisted, that epidemiology was "tracing the chain of infection." Furthermore, what right did I have, coming from the wealthy United States, to advise Eastern Europeans to avoid riding in automobiles, eating chocolate and meat, and smoking cigarettes?

His vehement attack on my presentation apparently led to my being invited, along with Donald Reid from the U.K., to participate in the "committee meeting" after the first day's adjournment. Completely puzzled about the "committee's" function, I learned upon arrival at the meeting place that our small group was assigned to formulate a statement that would reflect the discussions at the week-long meeting. No progress in that direction became evident at our Monday, Tuesday, or Wednesday early evening sessions, and I was becoming annoyed at missing the social events that were occurring during the meeting times. Things ended happily, however, on Thursday afternoon when the Russians brought to the meeting a brief statement attesting, in effect, to the virtues of motherhood and the joys of apple pie. Upon our prompt agreement with that noble pronouncement the Russians produced a huge box of chocolates. Seeking appropriate reciprocity I rushed to my room to fetch the bottle of bourbon which I had been carrying unopened to that time. Thus we celebrated our new East–West diplomatic agreement with chocolates and bourbon. Subsequently, I realized that my speech had no effect on the Russians.

Another episode at that 1959 Prague meeting, this one at the Thursday evening banquet, added to my education in international scientific diplomacy. A group of us were enjoying a balcony table overlooking a huge gymnasium where the recent medical school graduates were dancing in celebration of their becoming physicians. Suddenly and unexpectedly the Czechoslovakia Minister of Health, a defrocked Catholic priest who as an official in the communist regime still insisted on wearing his collar, joined our table and sat next to me. He immediately inspected the wine bottle labels; then he summoned a waiter and spoke to him rather sharply, whereupon the waiter took all the bottles off the table and shortly reappeared with another set. Upon examining them I found that German wines had been brought to replace the original Czech wines. Knowing that the World War II bitterness between Germany and Czechoslovakia had by no means completely subsided, I expressed surprise that the Minister advocated German wine over Czech wine and asked him why he did so. He responded, "In politics do politics; when drinking wine, drink wine."

INTERNATIONAL CANCER CONTROL

Although joining Cruikshank, Pemberton, Willard, and others in what became the IEA was my first international health venture, long-standing cancer interests and more general epidemiological and public health concerns led me into other sectors of the international arena. Having expressed interest in both international health work and cancer epidemiology I was invited in the late 1960s to join the U.S.A. National Committee for the International Union Against Cancer (UICC).

Participation in the UICC brought many opportunities to visit colleagues in other countries. That agency, which constitutes a major element of the non-governmental sector in international cancer control work, includes voluntary cancer societies, cancer research institutes, and cancer treatment establishments. A major aspect of the UICC's policy has been to encourage formulating and implementing national plans for cancer control. As chair of the UICC's National Cancer Plans project, which queried UICC members about their national situations, I participated in the 1988 decision to proceed with regional meetings to help formulate national cancer control programs, especially in developing countries where the incidence of cancer was now rising in a manner similar to what the developed nations had been experiencing for several decades. During the early 1990s I accepted responsibility for organizing on the UICC's behalf two regional meetings focused on national cancer control programs, one in Brazil for the South American countries and the other in Singapore for the Southeast Asian countries. The latter brought together thirteen cancer control and public health leaders from seven Southeast Asian countries, four from the United States, and two from Geneva. The conference participants had assembled data for each of their countries covering demographics; cancer in relation to other diseases; cancers in different sites; current resources for cancer control, including the national plan (if any), organization, and activities; and special problems. The conferees agreed that the role of cancer centers should be raising the visibility of cancer control; enhancing national pride; increasing morale among cancer control workers; and providing a center for cancer teaching and training, planning, conducting evaluation research, and treating advanced cancer cases. In summary, we thought that a cancer control centre should be a centre for cancer control, not simply a cancer hospital.

In both Brazil and Singapore, I advocated a public health approach to the regional cancer problems. That meant directing attention to the major cancer dangers that were affecting each region's people and aiming at prevention as the first priority. Program suggestions in those two areas included cigarette smoking control and developing cytology service (the Pap smear) for cervical cancer detection, a particularly important health problem in South America.

I learned, however, that those seeking cancer control in developing countries must combat the near-universal tendency for local experts to use whatever local resources are available for dealing with cancer first mainly for copying the high-tech approaches that prevail in the U.S. and other industrialized nations' medical centers. Young physicians from developing countries come to these centers to advance their expertise (particularly to learn new procedures) and then place their competence mainly at the disposal of cancer patients among the developing nation's "upper crust," the relatively few residents with high incomes. From the public health standpoint, which emphasizes total population health, resources for cancer control should be aimed principally at primary or secondary prevention of cancers that are jeopardizing health among the vast majority of the nation's population. That requires a very different message to those concerned with control than the one typically conveyed at high-tech medical centers located in New York, Boston, Los Angeles, or similar places.

I doubt that we made much headway during the UICC-sponsored Brazil and Singapore seminars in combating the message from institu-

tions in the United States and other highly developed nations that dissemi-
nate high-tech cancer diagnostic and treatment procedures. Experience
with cervical cancer in the U.S., where Papanicolaou developed the
cytological test, illustrates how much that single technique could, but
failed to, accomplish—even in a developed country. During the twenty-
five years immediately following World War II the negligence in applying
that technology allowed enormous numbers of Latin American women,
among whom the disease's relatively high frequency exacerbates the
problem, to die unnecessarily, whether in their native countries or as
immigrants to the United States.

   Another opportunity for participation in international cancer control
came my way when Mahler, then the WHO Director General, invited
me to draft a cancer control monograph for the WHO. I completed the
manuscript, which Anthony Miller, the Canadian epidemiologist and
consultant to the WHO, later employed as one element for a more
comprehensive WHO document.

CHINA

In 1977, Charles Grossman, a personal friend who has been active in the
U.S.-China Friendship Association, invited my wife and me to join an
American group visiting China. That was an exciting time because new
relations between our two countries, which President Nixon had initiated,
were opening longer opportunities for such travel. Americans had been
largely precluded from contact with one-fifth of the earth's population,
the Chinese people, for more than 25 years. That isolation resulted from
the U.S. commitment to the Chiang Kai-shek regime, which had retreated
from mainland China to Taiwan after the war against Japan, and the
subsequent struggle between the communist and the Chiang Kai-shek
forces. As a consequence of this international tension and isolation, we
had learned only vaguely of China's health situation.

   On that first trip to China and six succeeding ones Devra and I not
only saw much of that ancient, and now modernizing, nation but we also
became acquainted with several participants in its health achievements.
Among these, George Hatem, a Lebanese-American physician, had taken
the Chinese name Ma Haide when he joined the Chinese revolution
early in its course and became a key adviser to Mao on health matters
during the war years. Later Ma Haide organized the campaign against
Shanghai's prostitution activity and thereby overcame its longstanding
reputation as the world's syphilis capital. It has been alleged that the two
key features of that endeavor were rounding up the women and sending

them to the countryside for rehabilitation, and tracking down and executing the male pimps. Subsequently, Ma Haide initiated a campaign against leprosy. Hans Mueller, a German, Swiss-educated physician, also enlisted early in Mao's forces, but he preferred a military role in which he rose to command a medical contingent. In that capacity, as the struggle against the Japanese army ended in victory, Mueller encountered a Japanese nurse leader who, faced with surrendering her group either to Chiang Kai-shek's troops or to Mao's, decided on the latter because the Chinese Communist forces seemed to offer a better outlook for her nurses. That judgment brought her to Mueller, and events subsequent to that meeting eventuated in their marriage. Devra and I kept in touch through many years with George, Hans, and their wives, Sue Fei and Kyoko, and welcomed the Muellers to our home on their first visit to the United States. I recall Hans's response to my question after his first few days in this country, "What's the most striking thing to you in America?" "The number of fat people," he replied.

I was invited in 1979 to membership on the team that negotiated the first U.S.-China medical and health science exchange, a team led by Joseph Califano when he was U.S. Secretary of Health, Education and Welfare. Although the group included the long-time Florida Congressman Paul Rogers, journalist Art Buchwald, and other luminaries, the key discussions involved only four United States federal health officials, including Julius Richmond, the Assistant Secretary for Health and the leader of our side in the negotiations. I was the fifth and "outside" American participant. At our first joint session the Chinese appeared with more than a dozen health professionals. At the second session, however, only five Chinese came to the table; demonstrating the strong Chinese sense of reciprocity, they constituted our exact official counterparts: four from the People's Republic of China's national health agencies in Beijing, and one from a university in another major city. My opposite was Professor Wang, a Shanghai professor of public health. We became good friends in the course of our official discussions and accompanying social events, and we maintained contact for years thereafter.

The Chinese Health Minister, Chen Chi Xian, gave huge banquets for us. At one of them I happened to sit at a table where a Chinese participant challenged Paul Rogers to a drinking bout. The smaller and unfortunate challenger, however, was almost sinking under the table at the end of the meal while the larger-sized Rogers remained in good shape. At a subsequent affair and again seated with Rogers I observed the same Chinese man, then at a different table for ten Chinese men, visit his nemesis for another "bottoms up." After Rogers obliged him, however, a second man from the other's table walked over to confront

Rogers, and then a third, and so on. I worried that this friendly appearing chicanery was ominous until I saw how our Congressman was secretly managing to manipulate the three glasses that were in front of each of us. He would slip the powerful alcoholic Mai Tai drink, which was being used for the bout, into his half-empty large glass of orange drink and would then quickly replace the powerful liquor with contents from the third glass, which contained only water. The Chinese marveled at Rogers's seeming bottomless capacity for the one-against-ten drinking contest!

When Minister Chen brought a health delegation to the United States, I persuaded him to stop over in Los Angeles for a breather en route to the official Washington meetings and come to our home for an informal reception and dinner. Devra arranged a splendid affair on our patio, but it was marked by one untoward episode. A Chinese delegate with poor vision failed to recognize that a "blanket" covered our swimming pool. He stepped into the pool, fortunately at the shallow end. Pulled out and wet up to his waist, the unhappy medical scientist received what seemed to be a sharp reprimand from the Minister, evidently including instructions to return immediately to the hotel and not embarrass the delegation any more. Walking out with him, however, I suggested that he re-enter the house with me through another door and return to the party after a shower and change into a dry set of my clothes. The scheme worked well until a loud bang signaled his attempted re-entry from the house to the patio through a floor-to-ceiling window that he did not recognize as such. Again, fortunately, damage was minor, just a bruised forehead.

When I was in Beijing a short time later for a visit to a medical school, the translator for the Chinese ministerial delegation that had visited our home happened to encounter me in the hotel lobby. She expressed dismay that my presence was not known to the Ministry, and she indicated that the Minister would "want to do something." This "something" turned out to be a banquet for me the next evening with practically the whole delegation that had been in our home, and with the famous Peking duck as a special feature. In the course of the evening the Minister spoke jokingly about his colleague's mishap at our swimming pool, thus relieving my anxiety concerning that episode.

On another trip to China, while I was giving a lecture to a medical school class in Beijing, the rather elderly professor who had just introduced me suddenly remembered that he should have presented two items to the speaker. He hastened to hand them up to me while I was already lecturing: a huge cup of tea, which I placed on a convenient adjoining table, and a pack of cigarettes from which he had carefully tapped one partially out. His insisting in front of the class that I take the pack provoked a crisis for me that the students clearly recognized. My response was to throw the cigarette pack on the floor and stomp on it. While I was beginning to wonder whether the action might be a huge international blunder, the students applauded vigorously. I suspect they did so as much because they didn't like the professor as for the anti-tobacco message.

In 1990 the People-to-People Citizen Ambassador Program invited Devra and me to lead an epidemiology delegation to China. The delegation of 29 epidemiologists and six spouses and guests made visits to Beijing, Shanghai, and other cities, affording us an opportunity to learn about health problems in various parts of China, how they were being approached, and the status of epidemiology. We were also able to establish personal relationships with more Chinese epidemiologic colleagues.

During our visits to China, learning about the health progress being made in that huge country with such huge problems has indeed been inspiring.

NOT JUST WORK ABROAD

Visits abroad have involved family and friends extensively as well as professional activities. My two younger sons, while attending high school, accompanied me on trips to Europe, as Norman had done in 1957. Jack, my second son, traveled with me on a 1958 visit to Paris for an epidemiological conference, the usual tourist attractions of that city, and the World's Fair in Brussels. Our trip also included a stop in Leiden, the Netherlands, where I admired my first ergonomics demonstration—bricks that were designed for safe and efficient human handling rather than only for building. Stephen, my youngest, accompanied me to Prague when Karel Raska organized the 1959 Conference of Eastern European epidemiologists in that city and invited me to participate. We enjoyed Prague's splendor and many attractions and Stephen became well acquainted with Karel's son, Ivan. That family relationship was extended in 1995 when I took Stephen's son, Paul, to meet the third generation of Raskas in Prague and the Laursens, our family friends, on a farm near Copenhagen where it was a joy to see my grandson, a city boy, join in the farm routine.

Since our marriage in 1967 and move to UCLA, Devra has joined me at all IEA meetings, as well as on visits to China, Latin America, Africa, Japan, Australia, Indonesia, and several European countries. She is well known, especially to IEA leaders, and has welcomed to our home friends and colleagues from many parts of the world. In fact, not infrequently they greet me not with, "Hi Les, how are you," but with, "Hi, Les, how's Devra?"

On two occasions we visited Norman and his family in Lyon, France, while he worked at the International Agency for Cancer Research. On the first journey, we were privileged to watch our younger granddaughter, Sara, take her first steps across the room to me. In the 1980s Devra and I journeyed to another part of the world to be with Stephen and his family while they were on academic exchanges in Indonesia and Australia. We particularly enjoyed the home and family household that had been assigned to them in Indonesia.

In Japan I have appreciated meeting several of that country's famed epidemiologists, including Takeshi Hirayama, who joined the early group of investigators studying the effects of smoking. Devra and I have enjoyed travels involving professional work, tourism, and friends in several other Pacific Rim countries: New Zealand, Malaysia, and Papua New Guinea (PNG). Our trip to PNG in 1983 included meeting some new friends as well as John Lourie, a cousin of Devra's, who was conducting a nutrition project in the New Guinea mining area.

We met two of our newer friends, Ruth and Marshall Clinard, traveling up the Sepik River into Papua New Guinea where Marshall and I, two professors emeriti, volunteered to go crocodile hunting. The protocol for that adventure consists of entering a small boat launched from the river-vessel with a young Papuan guide, drifting quietly along the brush overhanging the river's edge, and watching for a pair of crocodile eyes at the water's surface. As the animal is about to pass, the hunter seizes the crocodile by the neck just back of the head and throws it into a barrel on the boat. Our guide explained that the trick is to judge how close the eyes are together. If they are far apart, the crocodile may grab you instead of you grabbing the crocodile, but if close together, the crocodile will be too small to impress the ladies back on the ship before it is thrown back into the river. When I recount that hunting expedition, my prey's size depends on whether I've had one or more drinks; if my wife is present she then typically interrupts me to insist that we have larger lizards around our house in Los Angeles (not true).

We observed two fascinating nutrition practices in PNG: one was raising crocodiles for meat commercially, and the other was using the sago palm tree for food. Papuans would chop the palm into small pieces, which they would then place in a fairly steep sluice through which they poured water to wash out the starchy nutritious material. The latter would be collected in a pail at the bottom of the sluice for food preparation, leaving the non-nutritious fiber behind on the sluice to be discarded. Some readers will recognize this process as the opposite of making potato latkes (pancakes) in which one presses the nutrient carbohydrate out of the potatoes and discards it with the fluid but retains the fiber for the pancakes.

When academic practice allowed me a five-month sabbatical leave during the 1977 spring and summer, Devra and I crafted a journey that mixed some professional engagements with travel to some new and some familiar lands, and that provided opportunities to see old friends and colleagues and make new ones. Our trip included London, where we gave a party for IEA friends; Toulouse, France, for a meeting on medical informatics; five weeks at the Rockefeller Study Center in Italy, to which scholars from various countries are invited to write or compose; to Israel for my first trip to that country where I enjoyed several informal professional visits including one with Michael Davies, who had participated in the first IEA meeting at Noordwijk; an international professional meeting in Tokyo prefacing a pleasurable visit to Kyoto, and then a somber one to Hiroshima; the USSR, where we were guests of the Ministry of Health; Latvia, where my mother's family originated; Lithuania, from which Devra's family had come to the United States; and Finland where we met Pekka Puska, epidemiologist at the National Public Health Institute, who was at that time initiating the subsequently renowned North Karelia cardiovascular disease control program, one of the earliest community-wide efforts to control that condition. During the summer months of the sabbatical we lived in Copenhagen, where colleagues provided me with an office to continue writing. As we enjoyed seeing many friends in that region and occasional visitors from the United States and elsewhere, the Scandinavian summer was a superb way to unwind before returning to UCLA responsibilities.

Over the years we have thus often blended (as many academics have the opportunity to do) professional work; personal travel; and opportunities to visit colleagues, family, friends, and projects. In our case that has involved traveling to more than thirty countries on six continents. As Devra sometimes pursued her own professional work at home, I undertook some of these trips alone, but whenever possible we made the journeys together. For example, early in 1997 prior to my lecturing in Alexandria, Egypt, at a public health institute, we traveled to Israel, where Devra's cousin hosted us. He took us by automobile, passing several Israel Defense Force military outposts taken from the Arabs in the 1967 war up to the Golan Heights. From the latter position we could see the outskirts of Damascus, about 20 miles away, and sense the continuing tension between Syria and Israel. Later, he drove us along the Eastern side of the Galilee, observing Arab and Jewish villages and the many posted mine fields. It was an opportunity to reflect on the regrettable cycle of violence that has plagued the area for so many years. In Alexandria we encountered Ramadan, the month-long period of daily fasting from dawn to dusk (which entailed no lunch after my lecture).

One of the dividends of my career in public health has been the personal aspects of international connections. Since Devra and I settled in Los Angeles, it has given us great pleasure to welcome scores of colleagues from many countries and their family members to our home, getting to know them in a more intimate context than at work. Their hospitality to us when we have traveled to their homelands has probably exceeded our own. We will never forget Helena Raska, the great pharmacology professor, who insisted on cooking a Czech meal for us in our home. Disregarding the summer heat she produced a marvelous pork roast, huge bread dumplings, which she sliced with thread, Czech style, and beets. Nor will we forget how the two eldest sons of Walter Holland, now in their thirties, first dangled their feet in our swimming pool. Or how Ken Tsuchiya, who would later become president of a major university in Japan, emerged for dinner in 1969 wearing his comfortable kimono. When I expressed admiration for it, he clapped his hands for his wife, Haru, to measure me. A kimono made by Haru arrived soon after, and I have worn that comfortable garment for dinner at home with Devra over many years.

Expansion of epidemiology internationally and its role in improving public health throughout the world has thus yielded great personal pleasures. I like to think that it has also provided one small link in developing the international community that the world's people are tending to become. The continuing regional conflicts and their tragedies could still explode into global disasters; devotion to health therefore demands that we struggle against combat as the solution to international health problems. After two great wars in the first half of the twentieth century we did seem to be taking effective steps toward a peaceful world where we could devote more energy to the advancement of health. As this was first written in September, 2002, that promise seemed to be dwindling again; now twenty months later it certainly has.

Just as peace creates the opportunity for improving health and a more livable world, achieving health creates the opportunity for a more enjoyable world and greater likelihood of peace. International health work has already succeeded in eradicating smallpox from the world. Further steps minimizing the threats to health are proceeding apace, although huge tasks remain in that regard, and new communicable diseases are appearing, notably HIV-AIDS.

REFLECTIONS ON INTERNATIONAL HEALTH

During the latter half of the twentieth century and now into the twenty-first, the developing nations have been struggling in the health arena mainly against the communicable diseases, whereas the developed nations have passed what is sometimes called the "epidemiologic transition," which means the border between dominance by communicable vs. noncommunicable disease. The noncommunicable conditions such as the cardiovascular diseases and cancer now are reaching into the developing nations as they become affluent enough to provide opportunity for increasing numbers of people to follow the causative lifestyle: more calories, especially from fats that people find tasty; less physical exertion; and smoking cigarettes. At first the more affluent people and then the rest of the population suffer from the chronic disease epidemics, and regrettably, we in the "advanced" nations have been doing very little to assist those who are starting to follow our lifestyle. We have remained passive about restraining those market forces from our own countries that are now exploiting people in the developing world, with severely adverse health consequences. As we begin to understand that the conditions of life largely determine the behavior that has led to the chronic disease epidemics, we discern that commercial interests often create and maintain disease-provoking conditions of life. Pushing tobacco and powdered milk exemplify the problem. Derek Jelliffe (deceased), a professor at the UCLA School of Public Health, and other public health leaders raised an international outcry against the Nestlé Company and so their sales practice regarding powdered milk, so adverse to health, was ultimately changed. We have not been so successful against the tobacco industry, which has become the paramount international, commercial health enemy. Attention must also be given to other companies that encourage products that are harmful to health, for example, those in the food industry that tout fatty foods to people who are ignorant of the consequences. Air pollution from industrial sources also knows no national boundaries, and thus is another situation in which some commercial interests must be combated in order to safeguard health.

Although international health work involves many facets, it should focus on raising the level of health in those parts of the world where poverty still prevails. That will involve not only positive aid, including public health components, but also combatting the economic forces from the industrialized nations that export health hazards during the recovery period.

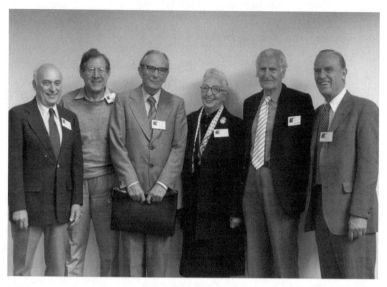

Founding participants of the International Epidemiological Association at the 11th Scientific Meeting of the IEA, Helsinki, Finland, August 1987. (L to R): Lester Breslow, Michael Davies, John Permberton, Joan Doll, Richard Doll, Carl Taylor.

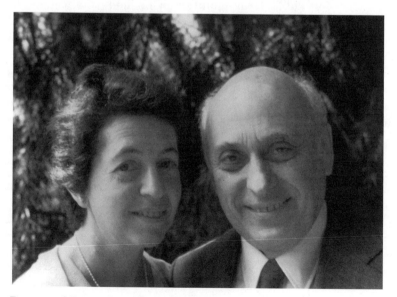

Devra and Lester Breslow, March 27, 1983, Los Angeles, California.

Academe

10

INTRODUCTION AND THE UCLA SCHOOL OF PUBLIC HEALTH

Formal university training for public health in the United States is usually said to have started in 1916 when the Rockefeller Foundation supported the Johns Hopkins University in establishing its School of Hygiene and Public Health. Although that was the first public health school in the modern sense, some training programs had been underway several decades earlier, first at the Massachusetts Institute of Technology (MIT) under the leadership of William Sedgwick. He recognized the need for joining biology with sanitary engineering science in response to the emergence of microbiology as the new basis for advances in public health. Subsequently, somewhat similar efforts to initiate training for public health work were undertaken at Harvard, Pennsylvania, Michigan, and Yale—particularly at the School for Health Officers which MIT and Harvard joined in founding. That venture collapsed after a few years, apparently because each university insisted on separately awarding its own degrees. The Hopkins pattern of education for public health ultimately prevailed. It emphasized biological science, as did Flexner's 1910 report, which laid the groundwork for medical education during the 20th century. By 1938 ten universities, both public and private, offered degrees in public health, among them the University of California at Berkeley. These programs of study involved varied relationships to the medical schools at the same universities. Tension between the two often arose during the formative years of institutional preparation for public health training and has extended to the present time, echoing controversy between medical practice and public health, mainly concerning the latter's role in providing and otherwise dealing with medical services.

Having initiated the Westwood campus in 1929, UCLA started its medical school immediately after World War II when Stafford Warren from Rochester, New York, was invited to become the founding Dean. Steven Goerke then moved from his post as Los Angeles City Deputy Health Officer to become chairman of Preventive Medicine in the new medical school. From that position he quickly established a Southern branch of the original University of California School of Public Health, located at Berkeley. Although the Dean at Berkeley, at that time Charles Smith, strongly resisted the effort to make the UCLA school autonomous, by 1961 Goerke had persuaded the UCLA Chancellor and the UC Board of Regents to establish a separate UCLA School of Public Health. It was pieced together from several existing elements on the campus including three biostatisticians on the Medical School faculty who received joint appointments in Public Health; five members, mostly nutritionists, of a Home Economics Department that was being dismantled; social scientists from other nonmedical departments; and an epidemiologist whom Goerke had brought from the City Health Department to the Medical School.

Through the 1960s the UCLA School of Public Health grew slowly, with Goerke as Dean concentrating at first on undergraduate education but moving steadily toward graduate professional education, and then essentially abandoning undergraduate courses. NIH funds provided research grants and some teaching support; the School's competence in obtaining such monies enhanced its national reputation as well as its work at UCLA. By 1968 Goerke had assembled a diverse faculty, though still in one department, which one member at the time described as a "mom and pop" operation. The School announcement for 1968–1969 actually lists 121 faculty members. Just twenty-eight of these, however, were tenured at UCLA and only sixteen of them had primary appointments in Public Health; the other twelve maintained their major affiliations in the medical, dental, nursing, and other schools on the campus. The School's tenured and other faculty members were distributed among eleven divisions: biostatistics, environmental and occupational health, epidemiology, behavioral sciences in public health, health education, infectious and tropical diseases, medical care organization, nutritional sciences, public health organization and administration, hospital administration, and international health. Those employed as lecturers or with other titles did much of the teaching; many of them did not qualify to become professors. Thus Goerke succeeded, with federal as well as state support, in developing a school that covered most aspects of public health, though rather thinly from the academic standpoint. It tended to be extensive horizontally rather than vertically. Faculty members were kept reasonably happy by the Dean's effective advocacy for the School and his personal leadership. Socializing at parties at his home was an important element of life in the School.

MOVE TO UCLA AND FIRST PERIOD THERE

I was recruited by Steve Goerke and Milton Roemer, a nationally leading public health figure then on the UCLA School of Public Health faculty, especially devoted to medical care and a long-time personal friend of mine. My arrival at the School in January 1968 was accompanied by considerable easing of my personal life, though with new challenges. I had completely ended my previous unhappy marriage and happily brought Devra, my bride of a few months, to a new life situation. I was also completely out of the stressful Reagan administration and into a totally new portion of my career, this time an academic one.

The only other professional opportunity I had considered when leaving the California Department of Public Health came when Mayor John Lindsay of New York City explored my becoming Commissioner of Health there. In many ways that possibility attracted me: leading a longstanding excellent and indeed famous Department, returning to the place where my father and many like him had started in this country, and working for a mayor with whose ideology I was comfortable. I don't know what Lindsay's decision might have been, but my decision not to pursue the matter probably mainly reflected my wanting to avoid repeating the Reagan experience because I wasn't too sure how long Lindsay would remain as mayor. Academe, on the other hand, suited my developing interests and appeared to be a good, stable place for the next part of a public health career.

In addition to building the School of Public Health, Goerke had continued in his position as chairman of Preventive Medicine in the Medical School. That dual capacity, however, did not seem very effective in bridging the underlying tensions between public health and medical practice that were reflected in academic life. After several outstanding medical leaders had taken prominent roles in the early development of public health including its University connection, considerable strain had grown during the first half of the twentieth century, particularly as public health moved to provide medical services for pregnant women and children without stringent economic barriers. Thus, in organized medicine's view, it began intruding on private medical practice. Physicians tended to resist whenever public health offered new medical services, such as screening for chronic diseases, or sought national or state programs to expand governmental assurance of people's access to medi-

cal services. In response, public health professionals began to regard
organized medicine as hostile to public health. In very recent times,
however, national and state public health and medical bodies have begun
to explore seriously how they can once again collaborate in advancing
people's health.

My coming to the School coincided with the arrival of Telford Work,
a laboratory-based epidemiologist. He proposed that the School separate
its members into two departments: one devoted to biological sciences
applied to public health that Work would lead, and the other concerned
with what administrative and social sciences could contribute to the field,
which I would chair. Although not enthusiastic about the idea, I did not
oppose it, feeling ambivalent about such an academic matter. The faculty
intensively considered Work's suggestion but finally rejected it. In retrospect I believe that was a wise decision because it would have impeded
a more coherent approach to public health into which the School has
evolved.

I settled comfortably into the School just as it was moving into the
Center for the Health Sciences where the medical, dental, and nursing
schools were located. Using data from the Alameda County studies that
I had carried with me from the State Department of Public Health
(though the continuing responsibility for the enterprise remained there),
I continued research work in addition to starting some teaching.

Having just come from general public health administration as the
State Public Health Director, rather than from another academic post
like most of the faculty, and encountering only Goerke and Roemer in
the School with practice experience similar to mine, I emphasized a
broad approach to public health in my teaching rather than a disciplinary
one. That emphasis involved some struggle against the university's predominant fostering of academic disciplines, which pervaded even professional units such as the School of Public Health where faculty from
several biological and social sciences had assembled. In a university like
UCLA, which prides itself on being a research institution, the Ph.D. is
an important focus. That fact, together with the relative newness of public
health as a field of professional study, encouraged the faculty to stress
typical graduate education based on disciplinary training rather than
professional education for public health. Peer reviews for academic promotion continue to give the greatest emphasis to research productivity.
Not much attention is given to practice, contrary to the situation in
medical schools where professional performance receives substantial
credit.

In spite of our disparity in precept, however, my colleagues welcomed
me and seemed happy to include another viewpoint. My considerable

research and several published papers while in the State Department of Public Health seemed to make me an acceptable academic. That background also greatly facilitated approval of my teaching concentration on public health practice. The difference in viewpoint, however, has never left my consciousness. I acquired a striking impression of how difficult teaching students to become public health professionals can be in a situation where individual academic disciplines weigh so heavily. Though multidisciplinary work became the byword, it seemed mainly a catch phrase to paper over the fundamental emphasis on the centrality of the disciplines.

Besides organizing new courses emphasizing public health practice for students I was also active in national and international public health activities, serving in 1968 on national health advisory bodies concerned with matters such as atomic bomb effects and health services research, and as President of both the American Public Health Association and the International Epidemiological Association. These latter responsibilities, which included being on the executive bodies before and after the presidencies, took me away from local academic work a good deal but did not seem to evoke faculty objection.

SOCIAL MEDICINE

Meanwhile, Goerke suffered an illness in 1970 that necessitated his relinquishing the chairmanship of Preventive Medicine in the Medical School; however he kept the School of Public Health Deanship. At that juncture Sherman Mellinkoff, Dean of the Medical School, invited me to succeed Goerke in that school while also keeping the professorship in the School of Public Health. As I plunged enthusiastically into the new responsibility my first action was to change the Department's name to Preventive and Social Medicine. That was consistent with what many people in preventive medicine believed at the time, namely, that we should combine the traditional preventive aspects of medicine with efforts to adapt medicine to current social needs.

We believed that medicine had become too highly focused on its high-tech, specialty components and was neglecting what Sigerist and others regarded as its being an essentially social endeavor to improve the people's health (Sigerist, 1943). Medical education was concentrating on producing narrower and narrower specialists who were applying biological sciences to the diagnosis and treatment of disease mainly as medical disciplines, but without sufficient consideration of what people needed overall for their health. It was diverging more and more from attending to that need in two important respects. One was intensifying specialist and sub-specialist training and according great academic prestige to those efforts, accompanied by academic denigration of the general physician, who was later to become known as family physician and primary care doctor. That tendency to emphasize the specialties highlighted the professional discipline rather than the patient. The other big deficiency in medical education was the failure, consistent with the attitude of most medical practitioners, to consider seriously how medical services could be assured to all people who needed them.

Those of us in social medicine thought that medical educators in the U.S. generally gave little or no attention to the problem of medical care to the underserved, that is, the many people who would benefit from it but could not obtain it. It was not just disagreement with medical school colleagues concerning national health insurance as the proposed solution to the problem, which many of us in preventive and social medicine advocated. We also observed that some medical care is good for health, some is harmful, and a substantial amount of it is just superfluous. Pursuing that observation alienated us professionally from some of our medical colleagues, on and off the campus. Departments of preventive and social medicine also sought to overcome the insufficient production of general physicians, a move in which they often joined the emerging forces toward family practice, and to expand academic medical services to underserved people. The latter effort attracted some idealistic medical students to preventive and social medicine.

At UCLA a few of us began emphasizing social medicine in that sense. A good opportunity arose in our collaboration with several medical and dental school faculty members to initiate the Venice Family Clinic. A largely UCLA-volunteer medical and dental-staffed clinic, this ultimately became a highly successful community operation. Devra and I recall pleasurably hosting a key development meeting for that venture in our home. The Venice Family Clinic typified the California movement for that form of medical service and became the largest community clinic in the nation, supplementing governmental medical care for the poor. It did so mainly by enlisting volunteer professional staff and establishing a more informal eligibility for services than governmental agencies could adopt. Because they have often become so effective, many such community clinics have been receiving governmental funds rather than such funds being allocated only to governmentally operated facilities for treatment of the poor. They have also become important venues for medical student education concerning the societal aspects of medicine.

In another social medicine venture C. Avden Miller, Vice-Chairman for Health Sciences at the University of North Carolina, and I organized in 1969 the Citizens Board of Inquiry into Health Services for Americans. With a Board representing a wide spectrum of American leaders including the Hon. David Bazelon, Chief Judge, U.S. Court of Appeals, Washington, D.C.; Einar Mohn, International Director, Western Conference of Teamsters; and Nathan Stark, Vice President, Hallmark Cards, we sought the voice of the consumer on medical services rather than giving the usual, exclusive attention to facilities, personnel, organization of services, and payment for them. By interviewing people across the country we found that "Americans are angry about health services . . . Consumers feel that they are locked in a system of health care that exploits them financially and leaves them powerless and at the mercy of health care providers. But we found that physicians, too, are angry and frustrated and concerned" (American Public Health Association, about 1971, but not dated, p. IV).

BECOMING DEAN OF PUBLIC HEALTH

Two years after I took up the Preventive and Social Medicine chairmanship, Goerke's health deteriorated further, forcing him to resign as the School of Public Health Dean. Following the usual national search, Chancellor Charles E. Young asked me to succeed Goerke as School of Public Health Dean. At that point I proposed to Mellinkoff that we amalgamate the Department of Preventive and Social Medicine faculty and other resources into the School of Public Health, which would then provide teaching and other input to the Medical School from the larger base. That followed a pattern established by the UCLA medical and dental schools in which the former taught basic medical sciences such as anatomy and physiology to the dental students. Mellinkoff agreed and asked me to continue serving on the Medical School Council to assure effective relationships.

Faculty in the School of Public Health were somewhat wary of my becoming Dean, one of them later informed me. They feared that I would be too strong, too heavy handed rather than fully respecting faculty views and bending to their desires. That may be a usual academic concern about someone coming into an academic leadership position from a career in a governmental bureaucracy where shared governance does not prevail, particularly as strongly as it does in the University of California system. In our case, however, the faculty was apparently even more worried about an outsider, and at least they knew me personally and as a current colleague.

The 15 to 20 years of early movement of people and activities between preventive medicine in the UCLA School of Medicine and the emerging

School of Public Health typified what several universities around the country were experiencing. Several public health schools grew out of similar academic medicine bases. At UCLA mutually supportive and respectful relationships prevailed among leaders of the two schools, though many medical school faculty members, like physicians generally, tended to express disdain for members of the medical profession who had abandoned individual patient care in order to devote themselves to public health. The feelings were reciprocal, though public prestige and recognition went largely to the providers and teachers of increasingly spectacular personal health services. The hostility seemed mainly inspired by medical practitioner antagonism to public health agencies because they were providing medical services for certain conditions and segments of the population, thus "intruding" on medicine's domain. Recently, an attitude shift toward greater collaboration appears to be occurring and will be discussed subsequently.

Two surprising events marked the first few months of my School of Public Health Deanship in 1972. The UCLA Executive Vice Chancellor, David Saxon, offered to increase the School's regular state-funded faculty positions by 50 percent, provided we systematically filled previous positions as well as the new ones with people who would qualify for regular university faculty appointments rather than using funds for "fill-in" teachers from around town who did not qualify for University appointment, as Goerke had been doing. That created the opportunity to build the School substantially, both in size and quality, and I eagerly took advantage of it.

The second event occurred at my home where I was hosting members of the Association of Schools of Public Health that happened to be meeting in Los Angeles that year. Bernard Greenberg, then Dean at North Carolina, approached me that evening saying that several deans were unhappy with the prospect next day of electing the person scheduled to be the Association's next President; they wanted instead to elect me. That was embarrassing to me on two obvious counts: first, my having just become a public health Dean, and second, what seemed like a conspiracy to empower me that was being orchestrated in my own home. Having known Bernie for some years, however, I trusted his insistence that he represented the overwhelming majority of members, and that it would be an appropriate and strongly supported step for the Association. I thus became the ASPH President as a newcomer to the organization. My major action in that capacity was my leading the search for an Executive Director for the Association. Fortunately that resulted in selecting Michael Gemmell, who had gained experience representing county governments in Washington, D.C. and who has served the Association very well for three decades. With his stewardship the Association has significantly strengthened and expanded the nation's schools of public health.

My initial aims as Dean of the UCLA School of Public Health were (1) to overcome the lingering extreme heterogeneity of the faculty and the failure to cover some major aspects of public health with regular, University-caliber faculty, and (2) to utilize Saxon's support for building a genuinely integrated faculty and a curriculum devoted to preparing students comprehensively for careers in public health. The circumstances and base for Goerke's founding of the School had brought several excellent professors onto the faculty but altogether too few and disparate to provide a cohesive, comprehensive approach to public health. Though my aims may have seemed mundane enough, both my naiveté and the University of California system presented difficulties in their achievement.

The strong power the faculty possessed in connection with administrative action, and particularly in the appointment of faculty, constituted one problem in moving ahead as I desired. It really was quite different from working in a state bureaucracy. Faculty strength in the governance system enhanced typical university professors' tendency and ability to replicate themselves not only in teaching students but also in faculty appointments in closely related fields. Our situation required my dealing with faculty eagerness to focus on building their own disciplines, which often seemed to me stronger than their allegiance to public health. The latter, of course, is essentially multidisciplinary and targeted broadly to the whole population's health. Academically, it entails bringing in expertise from several biological and social branches of knowledge—medicine, organic chemistry, bacteriology, sociology, statistics, nutrition, anthropology, and many others—but also melding them to focus on the community's health in order to train professionals and to advance knowledge for the field as a whole.

My own experience in local, state, and to some extent national and international governmental health work perhaps overly influenced my inclination to emphasize governmental activity as the core of public health work, and thus to believe that education for the field should stress helping students shape careers for that aspect of it. That view, I now realize, did not take into sufficient account the need to prepare young people for all the other ways that society has devised to improve the health of people—for example, teaching in colleges and elsewhere; research opportunities in various agencies; work in voluntary health organizations dedicated to controlling certain diseases; and nongovernmental agencies in local community, state, and national situations that provide all kinds of health services. Governmental health careers are crucial but not the only path to advancing public health.

My general intent was to shape the School into what seemed to me a logical organization encompassing faculty competence in the ways by which public health delineates and assesses problems: through epidemiology and biostatistics; and in the ways public health protects and improves population health, that is, by means of environmental, medical, and behavioral measures. Confronting the fact that the School had evolved into eleven divisions by the late 1960s under the influence of faculty seeking to replicate themselves in their disciplines, my objective was to build strength in the five specific, major fields and form corresponding faculty clusters as departments. For some components, for example, biostatistics, that posed no great problem because of the size and competence of its faculty and the general recognition of that public health field's uniqueness. However, many of the School's faculty members at the time had come from various other UCLA departments; some others were committed to their own disciplines and did not readily see themselves as fitting into a new paradigm. My difficulty was, of course, typical of what a newly appointed agency leader faces; he must deal with people in the organization who have been longer associated with it than he, and do not immediately share his view of the School's mission and the organization needed to accomplish it. Although some progress was made toward my objective during the 1970s when I served as Dean, substantial accomplishment came more than a decade later, during Abdelmonem Afifi's Deanship. A biostatistician, he became Dean in 1980 and with his leadership the School finally did establish five departments corresponding to the two diagnostic and the three therapeutic arms of public health. As noted earlier, it was probably fortunate that the earlier attempt to form two departments, one for the field's biological components and the other for the social and administrative components, failed. Although these two major aspects of science must be strongly represented in a school of public health, it seems preferable that they be integrated into such departments as epidemiology and health services. The School did manage to recruit several excellent faculty members in the 1970s who aided expansion of its teaching and research competence and attracted increasing numbers of first-rate graduate students.

Several programs established in Goerke's regime continued to flourish, for example, the one devoted to hospital administration. That program's vigorous enterprise attracted national recognition and linked the School into the local professional community, which provided great support for the entire school. Strength likewise grew in several other elements of the School.

I initiated two new features. In what came to be called affirmative action, universities were reaching out to students from socially disadvantaged backgrounds. That was particularly important in public health, which directed so many of its services toward overcoming health disparities and thus needed personnel who could relate culturally to minority groups. Proceeding in that direction we quickly discovered that such students, though qualified for admission, often required special help to succeed in the University environment with its special demands. To meet that need we organized a six-week orientation and introductory course that was offered just prior to the start of the formal, regular classes each year. I have been pleased over the years to meet graduates who took advantage of that special course and went on to excellent, sometimes academic, careers in public health. The second item was a course in writing that I persuaded a UCLA Professor of English to present in the School of Public Health. We encouraged all of our students to take that course because many situations in public health entail responsibility for good written communication, and students generally required improvement in that regard.

Devra and I greatly enjoyed entertaining new and older faculty members and students in our home. Small groups came to our dining room during the winter season and larger groups to our patio when warmer weather prevailed. That is, of course, what many deans, including me, regard as important for their schools and pleasurable for them as hosts.

SERVING AS DEAN

In addition to dealing with strategic academic issues and building and maintaining morale, being Dean also entailed a host of School administrative matters that extended broadly onto the UCLA campus and into the larger University of California system. The usual management tasks such as program development, personnel, and budgetary decisions were familiar from my prior experience in the California State Department of Health. The personal relationships there with staff and bureau chiefs that Halverson and Merrill had established, and I tried to emulate, provided experience for creating generally similar relationships between Dean and faculty and staff in the University of California system. As noted earlier, deans are considerably restrained by faculty power that the Board of Regents allocates, but in both governmental and university situations, the top official uses highly personal decision-making authority only on limited occasions; most decisions are formulated and measures for implementing them are established mainly through consultation among the parties. Several faculty members, who had longer experience in the

University of California system than I, gave me valuable advice in that sphere.

At the campus level deans are extensively involved in multischool program development and in reviewing and acting in situations where special effort beyond any one school is required. For example, Fred Rasmussen, Associate Dean of the Medical School, and I took substantial roles in developing the Jonsson Comprehensive Cancer Center (JCCC) at UCLA. This was one of several such centers that were established mainly in universities with support from the National Cancer Institute to pull together the several scholarly and service elements necessary for a comprehensive attack on cancer within an academic institution. They have become major foci of cancer research and improvement of cancer treatment around the country. Unfortunately, in my view, like the National Cancer Institute itself, the centers have not done enough toward cancer control in their communities, and my own performance as chair of the Chancellor's Advisory Committee for the JCCC proved not very effective in that regard. What the JCCC has done best, like most such centers, is to create a milieu that favors collaboration among various biological and clinical scientists working on several aspects of the cancer problem. Relatively little support has been devoted to stimulating or guiding community measures for cancer control, though in recent years the UCLA Center's unit devoted to Cancer Control and Prevention Research has been making considerable headway.

Another proposed UCLA Center, in which I became very involved, was aimed at the Study and Reduction of Violence, which ran into serious difficulty at its outset. Louis Jolyon West, a brilliant thinker and innovator as Director of the UCLA Neuropsychiatric Institute, led the effort to create that center. The venture reflected his own extensive experience and his profound interest in all kinds of human violence that has unfortunately continued to permeate the world. Bringing several campus elements into the enterprise, he sought a broad approach to the problem and particularly emphasized a potential biological basis for it. Regrettably, however, one of his first faculty recruits arrived advocating prefrontal lobotomy as one possible avenue for preventing violence. That surgical procedure was intended to separate one part of the brain from the rest in order to destroy a certain pathway in the brain's functioning and thus, he proposed, immobilize a tendency to violent behavior. The prefrontal lobotomy theory aroused intense opposition in Los Angeles, which had only recently experienced severe ethnic confrontation in which the alleged propensity of African Americans to violence had emerged as an issue. Such allegations stimulated fears in that community that the University might be contemplating brain surgery as a biological weapon in the local ethnic battles. The recently arrived faculty member had acquired a reputation in his previous position in Boston for pursuing lobotomy as a solution to the violence problem; it would have presumably entailed performing the procedure in Los Angeles on a highly disproportionate share of African Americans. His coming to the newly established Center evoked widespread opposition in the whole Los Angeles community and on the campus, where student demonstrations against his appointment and the Center itself attracted off-campus groups. As the situation became tense, Chancellor Young appointed me chair of a faculty committee to review the new Center. As a result of that tough assignment (and certainly other factors), the Center was not allowed to take root, a decision based both on its social implications and on evaluation of its biological potential.

Other activities on the campus were less onerous, for example, my serving on advisory bodies for (1) the Crump Institute of Medical Engineering, which assembled experts from the two fields for joint work on problems to whose solution both could contribute, (2) the Clinical Scholars Program, the UCLA element of a national endeavor by the Robert Wood Johnson Foundation to encourage young physicians toward research on medical services, (3) the UCLA Hospitals and Clinics, and (4) two searches for Dental School Deans.

One Friday afternoon, University of California Vice President for Finance, Chester McCorkle, telephoned me urgently requesting that I come to his Berkeley home the next day to discuss a critical matter affecting the three new U.C. medical schools that were then being established on the San Diego, Irvine, and Davis campuses. That Saturday morning McCorkle asked me to chair a system-wide faculty committee to formulate a plan for hospitals that would serve as clinical training resources for students in these new medical schools. The two U.C. system medical schools then existing at San Francisco and Los Angeles utilized University hospitals on their campuses. The three new Deans expected similar facilities for their schools. Alarmed at being responsible for financing and administering three new hospitals, the University administration wanted some alternate recommendation that it could present to the Board of Regents. Evidently the University leadership had been carried along in the wave of enthusiasm during the 1950s and 1960s to establish more places for training physicians, but without adequately considering how their essential clinical facilities would be provided. It had been evident for years that California suffered from a hospital bed surplus. The Kaiser Health Plan had demonstrated that good medical care could be provided with substantially fewer than the traditional number of hospital days per admission, and that idea was spreading in California, which was using fewer hospital days per 1,000 people than the national average.

I agreed to take on the obviously difficult task provided the U.C. administration would use the opportunity to establish a permanent Strategic Planning Team for the Health Sciences; McCorkle readily assented to that proposal. Excellent faculty members from several campuses came onto the Team and worked energetically, reviewing the various possibilities for providing the necessary clinical training facilities to which the University was now committed. In each case we considered the prospect of using hospitals then being operated by the respective county governments, the Veterans Administration, or others in the community, in addition to the possibility of building and administering new University hospitals. The Board of Regents, to whom the U.C. administration asked that I personally present our Team report, adopted our recommendation that all three new medical schools use existing clinical resources rather than building new campus hospitals. That report and the Regents' action in approving it did not endear me to the three disappointed medical school deans. The decision, however, has worked well from the State's hospital bed standpoint, and the medical schools seem not to have suffered significantly.

ACTIVITIES OUTSIDE THE UNIVERSITY

Two encounters with the hospital world beyond the University of California system illustrate how a public health school dean can become involved in health affairs outside academe. My service on the Los Angeles City Medical Advisory Committee included investigating arrangements at the scores of hospitals, many of them quite small proprietary facilities, that the city Council had officially designated to provide emergency medical services. The hospitals insisted that they were providing excellent services evidenced, they claimed, by the fact that they employed physician-trainees (residents) from the major local teaching hospitals for the night and weekend shifts when most emergency patients appeared. It seemed strange to me, however, that the hospitals agreed to accept such patients for only an eight dollar fee, until I learned during the investigation that the hospitals paid the young physicians a fifty dollar bonus for every patient that they decided should be "worked up" for admission. This, of course, brought the hospital considerable money for an inpatient stay. Exposure of that situation with its corrupting three-party win, including connections to local politicians, facilitated developing the area's currently excellent (though overworked) emergency medical service.

The second episode occurred during the 1970s when proprietary hospitals were making considerable headway toward becoming major players in providing inpatient services for Californians, but clearly emphasizing their "bottom line" to the detriment of their services. They were pursuing a quite different orientation toward their roles than what we had long experienced with public and nonprofit hospitals, actions that provoked me to make some uncomplimentary public remarks about the hazard the proprietary hospitals represented. On one occasion a couple of their leaders visited me in the Dean's office, obviously to straighten me out. They insisted that I was completely wrong to hold hospitals responsible for things that happened in them. Didn't I know that everything in hospitals was done according to a physician's order? If I had any problem with performance in hospitals I should take it up with the physicians there, not with the hospital owners. After hearing the two visitors present that argument three or four times, I recounted to them my previous experience with that reasoning: the case made 35 years earlier by the brothel owners in Winona, Minnesota, who alleged that anything "bad" going on their houses must be due to "those girls." That analogy evidently caused my guests to leave, convinced that persuading me of my "error" was impossible.

Election in 1975 to the Institute of Medicine, National Academy of Sciences, (IOM) allowed for my participation in that body's activities, particularly those concerned with health promotion, disease prevention, and public health generally. When the IOM established a Division of Health Promotion and Disease Prevention in the late 1970s, I served in the development process as chair of its advisory committee, and subsequently as Founding Chairman of its Board. The latter, which appropriately included social and behavioral scientists as well as members with biological and medical expertise, has engaged in several highly productive endeavors for more than two decades. I also served another IOM venture, the Committee to Review Public Health, whose report, *The Future of Public Health,* stimulated the field to review itself critically and especially to deal with the IOM finding that public health in the United States was in disarray.

The nation's effort against AIDS, identified clinically only in the early 1980s, was gaining headway within a few years. As part of its contribution, the National Research Council established a Committee of the Behavioral and Social Sciences on AIDS research to assess and advance knowledge concerning those aspects of the epidemic. Apparently as an outreach to epidemiology, the Committee invited me to join. After a few meetings it appeared that the Committee was concentrating largely on the heterosexual spread of the disease, whereas epidemiological analysis indicated that the infection would soon travel from middle-class male homosexuals principally to low-income and minority elements of the population. It was becoming epidemic there among both males and females. That difference in judgment over where social and behavioral science should focus—on sex or class—evidently led to my very short term on the Committee.

The National Cancer Institute (NCI) offered other opportunities for me to join with social and behavioral scientists. For its Board of Scientific Counselors to the Division of Cancer Prevention and Control, on which I served as a member and then as Chair, the NCI assembled a multidisciplinary group with social-behavioral and preventive medicine expertise. Despite excellent Division leadership, that group has been precluded from adequately carrying out its mission, originally set by Congress, and has been dominated by NCI biological and clinical scientists. This dominant element insists that the Institute should limit itself to research and not wholeheartedly undertake cancer control activities even though they were specifically included in the Congressional mandate. Originally linking biological and clinical cancer research to cancer control apparently seemed desirable, but it has not favored cancer control. The situation may ultimately result, as I have long believed it should, in moving cancer control out of the NCI.

Periodic efforts to improve personal health services for the American people presented many situations in which academics could participate. For example, several of us joined the Committee of 100 for National Health Insurance to campaign for legislation that would assure medical care services for all Americans. Walter Reuther, longtime head of the United Automobile Workers, organized and led that effort. Although Reuther devoted his remarkable organizing talents, and the Committee added its members' vigorous support, the time was not right and the Committee had little impact. In a second venture aimed at improving the situation the American Medical Association joined with Senator Edward M. Kennedy, who had long advocated progressive health action, George Meany, then President of the AFL-CIO, and others to prepare a "Focus on Positive Health Strategies." It was exhilarating for me to appear at the group-sponsored conference along with Kennedy, Meany, and Tom Nesbritt, then President of the AMA, as a principal speaker emphasizing prevention. Again, however, and despite assembling people with widely varying viewpoints, not much seemed to be accomplished beyond agreement that prevention is important. A third recent thrust, which the American Public Health Association and the American Medical Association have undertaken, aims at encouraging medical and public health professionals and agencies to collaborate in community health projects. A New York Academy of Medicine panel, on which I served with several academics and practicing physicians, explored the rationale and prospects for that purpose. Subsequently hundreds of examples around the country have appeared, and groups in several states are pursuing further collaboration, for example, the California Medicine and Public Health Initiative. The time may be right for such rapprochement between medicine and public health and for overcoming their long estrangement; perhaps that path will begin with concrete local endeavors in which they come together. Major issues such as national health insurance on which there still appear no immediate prospects for agreement between the two will, of course, keep them divergent, but that should not impede progress on immediate steps toward specific health activities in which their different professional experience and situations can be merged.

THE UNIVERSITY PARADIGM

Each University of California professor, as in universities generally, is evaluated periodically by peers on the basis of teaching, research, and service. Promotion depends on rigorous investigation of the documentation related to all three spheres of academic activity.

Faculty members in the UCLA School of Public Health are expected to teach four courses, each extending about ten weeks per year. Besides the preparation and classroom appearances for such courses, individual counseling of students, review of student papers, and examinations must be provided. Faculty members also work personally with students pursuing studies leading to doctoral degrees. Often these students participate in a professor's research. Because my first four years at UCLA were so uneven, starting at the School of Public Health in the 1968 winter quarter, moving to the School of Medicine in July 1970, and then back to serve as Dean of Public Health from 1972 to 1980, my teaching responsibilities were relatively lighter than those of a typical faculty member. Increasingly over the years and extending to the present time my classroom teaching has consisted largely of invited appearances in courses for which other faculty members are mainly responsible. In addition I have participated on committees guiding and examining doctoral candidates (Ph.D. and Dr.P.H.), and taken primary responsibility for some. I have also joined in organizing and conducting courses aimed at teaching students about tobacco control, preparing entering students for graduate work, and interesting undergraduates in public health.

My California State Department of Health activities had included considerable research and publication, so that aspect of university work meant simply continuing what I was already doing. During the 1970s and early 1980s, for example, while in the School of Public Health, my publications included topics such as "Early Case-finding, Treatment and Mortality from Cervix and Breast Cancer" (1972); "Relationship of Physical Health Status and Health Practices" (1972); "A Quantitative Approach to the World Health Organization Definition of Health: Physical, Mental and Social Well-being" (1972); "Radiation Risk of Mammography" (1976); "Life-time Health Monitoring Program" (1977); "Risk Factor Intervention for Health Maintenance" (1978); "Persistence of Health Habits and Their Relationship to Mortality" (1980); "The Challenge to Health Statistics in the Eighties" (1981); and "Patient Education in Historical Perspective" (1985).

The service component of the university triad strongly attracted me and kept me alert to what was happening in the public health field outside academe. If the School were to prepare students and conduct research that would help solve society's health problems, it seemed crucial that both faculty and students gain intimate knowledge of current issues by actual public health work, just as medical students and their teachers provide actual service for patients. To that end I took advantage of opportunities for participating in all three phases of public health: medical, environmental, and behavioral, and tried to engage other faculty members similarly. For example, on the medical service side, California trade unions in the late 1960s became sensitive to the fact that approximately $750 million each year was going toward health insurance premiums for more than 1.5 million workers and their family members. Trustees of the health and welfare funds making the payments became concerned that the health plans were not improving as rapidly as their costs were rising. Faculty members on the University of California campuses in Los Angeles and Berkeley who were interested in how such expenditures were affecting health care held conversations that resulted in the California Council for Health Plan Alternatives. The Council initiated a project to develop a health plan grading system. That project, on which I served as Director, eventuated in a system that allocated points for the extent to which a health plan met specific criteria pertaining to administrative arrangements, coverage of family members, scope of benefits, provisions to assure quality of care, out-of-pocket expenditures, and premium costs. The system was applied in a pilot operation to ten California health plans and the results were published without identifying the plans. The project report, "Health Plan Grading System," published by the Regents of the University of California, may have played some role in furthering the systematic evaluation of health insurance plans in California and elsewhere.

The environmental health field also offers many opportunities for public health faculty to join community endeavors at local and state levels. The Santa Barbara County Health Officer, for example, called upon two of us in the UCLA School of Public Health—John Froines as a toxicologist and head of the Environmental and Occupational Health Center and me—to provide technical assistance when he encountered a difficult situation. Several County residents were insisting that a dump operating in their neighborhood was causing highly offensive odors and disease and should therefore be closed. The Health Officer requested that Froines and I join a committee to determine whether the dump was actually causing any disease. Although our investigation and report disclosed no evidence of a specific disease caused by the malodorous situation, we did not defend the dump and pointed to the considerable discomfort and long-term hazardous potential. Subsequently, the County Board of Supervisors decided to close the dump, evidently responding primarily to general public pressure and not our report.

My early State Department of Health air pollution work probably served as the basis for my appointment to a term on the Medical Advisory Committee to the California Air Resources Board, the body responsible for controlling air pollution. Initiated in the early 1960s, the state's program has vastly reduced the toxic substances that people take into their lungs. As the risk declines and the immediate irritating effects bother people less, industry appears emboldened to oppose the increasingly tough standards necessary to achieve improved air, claiming great cost consequences. The task is thus by no means complete, and the effort to protect Californians against air pollution will evidently continue indefinitely as a struggle between the forces seeking greater health protection and those seeking to minimize industry's expenditures, a struggle in which the Air Resources Board serves as the principal battleground. Balancing the estimates of reduced risk and increased dollar cost, both socially necessary considerations, is a difficult task. The United States has essentially copied the original California air pollution control plan and has charged the Environmental Protection Agency with responsibility for setting and enforcing nationwide standards. The issue now is whether state or national standards will prevail; some states seek greater protection than the national ones specify. We are at least fortunate in a democracy that the struggle proceeds largely in open meetings, public documents, and with free speech.

Asbestos exposure became highly visible on the national environmental health scene when studies revealed that it caused a vast amount of disabling and fatal lung disease. The asbestos experience typifies the growing recognition during the twentieth century's later decades that

adverse health consequences have flowed from the uncontrolled industrial development during the first half of the century. As steps were being
taken to remedy the asbestos situation, another question arose: Does
non-occupational exposure cause similar harm? The National Research
Council responded by establishing a Committee on Non-Occupational
Health Risk of Asbestiform Fibers, which I chaired.

We determined that non-occupational exposure to asbestiform fibers
in air presents a risk to human health, the extent of which is highly
uncertain. As evidence for that conclusion we cited several items including the observation of an excessive incidence of mesothelioma and other
abnormalities known to be caused by asbestos among household contacts
of asbestos workers (Committee on Non-Occupational Health Risks of
Asbestiform Fibers, National Research Council, 1984).

On the third avenue of public health endeavor (favorably influencing
health-related behavior), social and behavioral scientists now typically
lead the way. Historically and to the present day, however, public health
physicians have recognized its significance and have joined or have even
been leaders in the movement. As emphasis on health behavior has
increased, public health physicians in academe have played substantial
roles in studying what particular features of behavior—smoking, inadequate exercise, poor nutrition, and the like—harm health and in advocating healthful behavior.

Upon coming to UCLA I was quickly drawn into local American Cancer
Society activities, having participated for years in that organization's state
and national programs. Major efforts of local chapters have been directed
toward educating the public about cancer, especially its causes; how to
prevent it; the importance of early treatment; provision of services to
cancer patients to augment medical care; and raising funds for the Society. From 1975 to 1985 I helped lead these efforts in the organization
known as Community Cancer Control/LA.

Taking advantage of some new federal funds allocated to health promotion, a few other UCLA faculty members and I developed an inner
city council for that purpose. We settled on South El Monte, a community
of about 20,000 largely poor, Latino residents near the center of Los
Angeles. Beginning with a Steering Committee composed mainly of professionals serving the community but including some from local governmental agencies, the design included a Board consisting of grass-roots
people who gradually took over leadership of what became the Health
Promotion Council. The Council saw the health problems not as immunizations and Pap smears, which the health professionals emphasized, but
as gangs, violence, and drugs. The Council then convened fiesta-like
affairs with health messages that seemed more successful than the previ-

ous rather formal meetings. The switch in empowerment engendered tension with some local health professionals who did not relish "their" community being labeled as a hotbed for gangs, violence, and drugs, which the new agenda brought by rank-and-file residents implied.

This account of one academic's experience merely suggests the nature and range of situations in which public health school faculty members can serve local, state, and national interests and remain alert to emerging health problems that a school of public health should consider for research and teaching, the other two faculty responsibilities. Ending a public health physician career in such a stimulating atmosphere surrounded by vigorous younger faculty and students has been very satisfying and I am grateful for having had the opportunity to participate in academic public health.

Reflections and Recommendations

11

I n concluding this book it may be appropriate to mention some
reflections based on a sixty-five-year career as a public health
physician.

TURN OF THE CENTURY

At the end of the twentieth century public health had much to celebrate.
Smallpox, the scourge that devastated mankind for many centuries, had
been eliminated. That accomplishment reflected years of intensive effort
led by public health workers who narrowed its transmission to smaller
and smaller areas by erecting barriers of vaccinated people. Poliomyelitis,
another frightful disease, is now being attacked the same way with success
already throughout North and South America and most other parts of
the world. Measles is next on the list. Striking reduction of most major
communicable diseases, in fact, has largely freed people from the major
maladies that disrupted their lives a hundred years ago.

That accomplishment, though still incomplete and to be pursued
more fully, deserves accolades for being principally responsible for length-
ening the average life in the United States from 47 years to 77 years.
That was the first era in modern public health.

At the mid-century point, epidemiologists began to uncover the predominant causes of the new health problems, the chronic, noncommunicable diseases. Disclosing the factors responsible for these conditions
swept away the notion, still prevalent about 1950, that they were due to
senescence or natural processes of aging. It also made their prevention
possible by controlling tobacco use, fatty diet, and high blood pressure

and by expanding exercise. The tremendous reduction of the chronic disease burden by acting on that knowledge during the latter half of the century has not only facilitated the continuing increase in longevity, but has also relieved people of the considerable misery those conditions carried. That was the second era in modern public health.

Among these strides forward an important component has been advancing improved and new concepts of how to minimize disease and advance health. For example, the idea of secondary prevention of chronic disease (i.e., the discovery of such disease early in its course) often permits effective intervention that prevents later consequences that were formerly called "degenerative disease." Primary prevention, that is, the avoidance of disease altogether is, of course, always preferable. Another concept is expressed in the Institute of Medicine's statement of Public Health's mission: assuring "the conditions in which people can be healthy." That declaration recognizes the importance of identifying conditions—even general conditions and not just exposure to specific biologic, physical, or chemical agents—that are responsible for ill health, and attacking those underlying conditions. Thus, for example, we are achieving control of much disease by reducing access to tobacco smoking, a social condition, without knowing the precise chemicals or particles in the smoke that initiate the pathology. Further health advances depend to a considerable extent on our ability to identify the conditions that lead to poor health or good health, and supporting those that favor the latter.

As we enter the twenty-first century, we have been so successful in overcoming disease that the prospect of achieving health in an even more positive sense has arrived for increasing numbers of people. To describe the move in that direction the Ottawa Charter definition of health may be appropriate: health is a resource for everyday life. No longer do we only combat disease; now it is possible to seek or maintain the competence for what one wants to do in life—climb mountains, play cards, attend the opera, or whatever. To do so requires some capacities, for example, physical stamina, memory, vision, and hearing. Thus, we are currently entering a third era in health: the pursuit of health itself.

THE BREADTH OF PUBLIC HEALTH

Most people apparently think of public health as concerned with controlling epidemic disease, sanitizing the environment, and providing to vulnerable segments of the population certain medical services, especially these involved in maternal and child health. They have been the major and the most visible aspects of the public health field until relatively recent years and are still important components of its responsibility. Dealing with HIV-AIDS, or SARS, for example, receives considerable public attention; and whenever an upsurge of any communicable disease occurs, people tend to look to the health department.

Most of the time, however, things are rather quiet on those fronts and public health appears to be inactive, except insofar as the public regards tax-supported medical services as a part of public health. Actually, of course, health departments are constantly active: keeping track of births and deaths; practicing routine communicable disease control measures such as immunizations; maintaining surveillance of environmental sanitation and correcting deficiencies; inspecting hospitals, nursing homes, and other facilities to assure their safety; and myriad other duties.

These activities, however, are so below the news media horizon that they attract practically no attention except when, as at present, they are directed toward the threat of bioterrorism or some other situation in which the public is intensely interested. Generally, most federal, state, and local legislators view the public health department as just another bureaucratic agency that can be summoned in case of some emergency. Maintaining its readiness, even for such an event, is just another place to cut public expenditures—until an emergency actually occurs. Lack of immunization, failure to follow up tuberculosis cases, the epidemic of obesity and diabetes, and dozens of other health issues do not constitute such an emergency. That attitude has led to several cuts in allocations for public health, resulting in poor salaries, lack of positions and failure to fill even those available, thus weakening the basic structure of public health as well as restraining its expansion into needed areas. These include a whole new set of endeavors to deal with tobacco use (for which even specified funds have been misallocated to other purposes), excessive alcohol use, obesity, and sedentary life style, all of which lead to diabetes, heart disease, lung cancer, and other current significant diseases.

The much-needed public health approach to these problems requires epidemiological investigation of the conditions responsible for them; seeking correction of such conditions as dumping market-excess fats on school children, licensing excessive numbers of liquor stores, and failing to provide exercise facilities; and then monitoring the effectiveness of actions taken.

Thus far this chapter has focused on typical, essential state and local health department functions. Opportunities abound for expansion to maintain and improve health, for example, in nutrition, assuring adequate safe water supplies, training for exercise, research on the effectiveness of medical services, and numerous other situations. Federal public health leadership and support of such functions, as well as funding health research, has become a vital element in American public health. Furthermore, various governmental agencies—mental health, air pollution control, highway safety, water works, and many others—have been allocated responsibility for specific aspects of health protection. All of them are "ways in which society organizes to maintain and advance health," that is, public health; and they must be supported as public health endeavors.

Beyond governmental activity our society has fostered many ways to maintain and improve health. Prominent among these are voluntary health associations devoted to controlling cancer, heart disease, lung disease, diabetes, and other highly significant conditions through research, professional and public education, and service projects; foundations that support research, education, and demonstration projects; and community organizations that provide clinical services, education, and other means to improve health in their neighborhoods.

The entire array of these governmental and nongovernmental agencies and their activities thus constitute public health in the United States. Recognition of this breadth of organization and collaboration among its elements is essential to achieving the maximum from public health.

THE NEED TO POPULARIZE FOCUS ON POPULATIONS

Because people still tend to think of health care as medical and related service for disease problems in individuals, it is vitally important to make clear the role of public health: to improve health in populations. The goal is to maximize the health of communities: international, national, state or provincial, regional or local.

Any public health agency may concentrate its effort on a certain population. Within that group the agency may choose to focus a part or its total activity on some especially vulnerable segment of the population, for example, low-income people, those socially disadvantaged by ethnicity or other features of their lives, children, or the elderly. Because people tend to be unfamiliar with what the whole of public health does, it has become extremely important for public health to speak out much more vigorously concerning its role, aims, and achievements. Those who receive or see someone else receive a useful medical service appreciate what has been accomplished, but they generally do not know what public health does for them and all others in the community because such activity is taken for granted and escapes notice. If public health is to gain public support, it must strongly present a better account of itself.

As a part of thus promoting public health, its leaders must also take a more active part in the policy fray. They should not simply accept whatever legislators and government executives assign to them; their duty is to help formulate the health policies and programs for the entire population that they serve. That means vigorously espousing what they see as necessary to protect and advance people's health by becoming personally acquainted with the political leaders and their staffs in their communities, making themselves known as reliable sources of knowledge and insight concerning health issues, and lobbying for public health interests.

REGULATION OF PRODUCTION AND MARKETING

Our society is based on the production and marketing of goods and, more recently, of services. These processes sustain the economy and the livelihood of people in the society. Over the past couple of centuries, however, we have learned that these activities can entail some harm to health.

In fact, the unhealthful conditions in factories, including child labor, physical hazards in work, and poor wages stimulated efforts to protect health by establishing the public health movement as a part of the general social reform that was responding to the living and working conditions that prevailed during the early days of industrialization. Because of the tendency to curtail production costs by not spending the money necessary to maintain healthful working condition, it has been necessary to keep up the social action to attain and preserve such conditions. That action has taken the form of organizing workers into unions that can bargain for improved conditions, and rules and regulations adopted by the legislative and judicial branches of government. These are elements of public health's mission to "assure the conditions in which people can be healthy"; thus public health leaders generally strongly support these efforts, both by unions and by government, to seek healthful conditions of work. In the economic cycles wherein either political forces that favor cutting production costs or those favoring occupational health protection gain ascendancy, public health interests are at stake and should be pursued. In these earliest years of the twenty-first century in the United States, we are encountering a substantial dip in the cycle, manifested by attacks on regulations that safeguard health not only in the workplace but in the environment as a whole.

Marketing of goods and services may also involve harm to health. Although we maintain the principle of freedom to engage in trade as a major feature of our society, we have also come to recognize that some marketing practices are harmful to health. An outstanding example is the case of cigarette sales. Strong public health efforts have partially succeeded in turning back the tobacco industry's campaign to market cigarettes. That experience, together with overcoming aggressive sales of powdered milk to be mixed with polluted water, and other similar endeavors, points the way toward countering the marketing of products that cause health damage. Some aspects of the food industry, the drug industry, and the liquor industry—including their retail outlets—deserve similar public health attention. For example, the proliferation of liquor stores that promote sales in neighborhoods that are especially vulnerable to health harm should be curtailed. Again, ferreting out the facts, and then securing public and political support for desirable action are necessary for effective action in such situations.

While we abhor the unhealthful conditions that prevailed during the early period of industrialization and take pride in having overcome them to a considerable extent, the struggle against the harmful effects of production and marketing practices—like the struggle against the communicable diseases—seems never-ending.

PUBLIC HEALTH AND MEDICINE

Although public health emerged in considerable part, especially in its scientific base and technical aspects, through the leadership and support of progressive-minded physicians, relations between medicine and public health have not always been amicable. Society long ago established two arms for health: one for seeking conditions that protect and advance health in the whole population, and the other for care of individuals who fall sick. Because of their social value society supports training of practitioners for both arms, recognizes their professional status, and economically supports their efforts. The two arms are often linked, for example, in immunization of people against communicable diseases and in cancer control.

Nevertheless, from time to time substantial tension has arisen between medicine and public health, largely because the two professional groups have differing commitments. For example, public health practitioners have sought to assure access to clinical services for disadvantaged segments of society, when necessary, as governmental enterprises. That happened in the case of maternal and child health services when Congress passed the Sheppard-Towner Act in 1921. Such actions have provoked opposition by medical associations, which tend to see all clinical services as the province of private medical practitioners. Some medical leaders have also fought against the insistence of public health practitioners on high standards for governmental medical services, for example, in the California Crippled Children's Service. Meanwhile, some public health practitioners have resented the favored position of medical practitioners with respect to income, social prestige, and the political power they exercise over public health; they also criticize the guild-like characteristics of organized medicine.

Recent changes in the areas of conflict between medicine and public health, however, may open the window for fuller collaboration in the near future. One such trend is the growing perception that medical and related services are entering a crisis with respect to their cost, and the seemingly greater acceptance of governmental intervention; organized medicine may be needing allies. Public health may be receiving some relatively greater social recognition, for example, in the struggle against bioterrorism. These perceptions may just be straws in the wind, but they may indicate a beginning shift in relations.

One definitely hopeful sign is the development across the country of deliberate efforts to foster collaboration, as in the medicine–public health initiative. Certainly both health arms of society could more effectively fulfill their missions by greater collaboration and by minimizing the tension between them.

EDUCATION FOR PUBLIC HEALTH

Although education for the field started as training for health officers, it has veered considerably from that sole intent. Recognition has grown that the field requires an array of specialists: epidemiologists, biostatisticians, environmental health experts, behaviorists, service administrators, and others in order to carry out the mission. Hence, schools of public health and other training resources have developed programs to educate such specialists and to conduct research in the field's various scientific and professional areas.

That trend has drawn teachers and students into the public health training enterprise with backgrounds in the many areas of knowledge that are related to what public health does. Thus individuals with graduate degrees in mathematical statistics, social sciences, biological sciences, administration, and other disciplines have been appointed to faculty positions in the academic institutions that provide education for public health work. As people from these several disciplines have entered such institutions, they bring little or no experience in actual public health work, but they carry a strong commitment to the disciplines instilled in them by their training and experience in academe. That has generated a tendency among public health academics simply to replicate themselves, rather than to prepare students to work in public health. Those few faculty members capable of training leaders in the totality of public health, for health officer and other leadership positions, are now vastly overwhelmed in numbers. Influenced strongly by academe itself to advance the disciplines, schools of public health tend to obscure and, in effect, denigrate, teaching public health as a whole enterprise.

One evidence of this tendency is the fact that schools of public health in their doctorate programs emphasize the Ph.D. degree while the Dr.P.H. languishes. Public health training has thus become more graduate education than professional education. From time to time efforts are made to strengthen the Dr.P.H. program in various schools, but the strong pressure on faculty in the country's major research universities and that faculty's own training generally prevail. Most schools make a point of requiring students to do a field project in some public health agency, for "exposure" to public health, but too often these projects relate mostly to the academic concerns of their faculty advisors who themselves usually have little interest and no experience in working in the field.

A result has been that many public health officerships and other key administrative positions in health departments and other public health agencies are unfilled or staffed by people with inadequate training. Also, because of the tremendous need for training for public health work, more than forty institutions of higher education that are not yet capable of developing a school of public health have initiated more limited programs of training for work in the field.

When approached on this matter, faculty members often respond that public health positions do not pay enough to attract highly qualified applicants. That certainly is a part of the problem. Apparently it must be attacked on both sides: training and employment. An important feature of that attack consists of vigorously espousing what public health does in order to gain the necessary public support.

PERSONALLY SPEAKING

The opportunity to participate in public health has filled my years with exhilarating activities. Knowing that the field as a whole has been contributing so much to people's lives has tremendously invigorated my commitment to public health.

Preparing for and entering that area of work during the Roosevelt progressive-spirited era and pursuing it under the Earl Warren–Pat Brown leadership in California added zest to my career. Closing in academe at UCLA has added another special opportunity.

I regret that so many of my younger colleagues have been compelled to work under the far less propitious circumstances that dominate the current national and state scenes. However, this is only one phase of social evolution. Better times and new advances in health will come.

References

American Public Health Association 1970. Health Crisis in America. American Public Health Association (about 1971). Heal Yourself.

Auditor General, State of California. (1975). *Report of the auditor general on the Department of Public Health*. Sacramento, CA: Author.

Beers, C. (1921). *A mind that found itself* (5th ed.). Garden City, NY: Doubleday.

Belloc, N. B. (1973). Relationship of health practices and mortality. *Preventive Medicine, 2,* 67–81.

Belloc, N. B., & Breslow, L. (1972). Relationship of physical health status and health practices. *Preventive Medicine, 1*(3): 409–421.

Belloc, N. B., Breslow, L., & Hochstim, J. (1971). Measurement of physical health in a general population survey. *American Journal of Epidemiology, 93*(5): 328–336.

Berkman, P. F. (1971). Measurement of mental health in a general population survey. *American Journal of Epidemiology, 94*(2): 105–111.

Berkman, L. F., & Syme, S. L. (1979). Social networks, host resistance, and mortality: A nine-year follow-up study of Alameda County residents. *American Journal of Epidemiology, 109*(2): 186–204.

Boas, E. (1947). *Chronic disease, New York Academy of Medicine, Committee on Medicine and the Changing Order: Medical addenda.* New York: The Commonwealth Fund.

Bosch, X. (2003). *Archie Cochrane: Back to the front.* Barcelona, Spain: Catalan Institute of Oncology.

Breslow, L. (1947). *Chronic disease in the modern public health program.* California's Health.

Breslow, L. (1950). Multiphasic screening examinations—an extension of the mass screening technique. *American Journal of Public Health, 40,* 274–278.

Breslow, L. (1951). Senescence, chronic disease and disability in adults. In K. Maxcy (Ed.), *Rosenau's preventive medicine and hygiene* (7th ed., pp. 720–755). New York: Appleton-Century-Crofts.

Breslow, L. (1955a). Industrial aspects of bronchiogenic neoplasms. *Diseases of the Chest, 28,* 421–430.

Breslow, L. (1955b). The epidemiologist looks at smog. *Public Health Reports, 70,* 1140–1142.

Breslow, L. (1956a). Newer concepts in chronic disease. *Journal of the American Medical Association, 161,* 1364–1368.

Breslow, L. (1956b). *Chronic illness in California: California's health.* Berkeley, CA: Department of Public Health.

Breslow, L. (1957). Uses and limitations of the California Health Survey for studying the epidemiology of chronic disease. *American Journal of Public Health, 49,* 168–172.

Breslow, L. (1968). Medical care and health education. *Public Health Reports, 83,* 791–795.

Breslow, L. (1972). A quantitative approach to the World Health Organization definition of health: Physical, mental and social well-being. *International Journal of Epidemiology, 1*(4): 347–354.

Breslow, L. (1972). Early case-finding, treatment and mortality from cervix and breast cancer. *Preventive Medicine, 1,* 141–152.

Breslow, L. (1976). Radiation risk of mammography: Another view. *Western Journal of Medicine, 125,* 495–497.

Breslow, L. (1978). Risk factor intervention for health maintenance. *Science, 200,* 908–912.

Breslow, L. (1981). The challenge to health statistics in the eighties. *Public Health Reports, 96*(3):231–236.

Breslow, L. (1982). Control of cigarette smoking from a public policy perspective. *Annual Review of Public Health, 3,* 129–151.

Breslow, L. (1985). Patient education in historical perspective. *Bulletin of the New York Academy of Medicine, 60,* 115–122.

Breslow, L., et al. (1977). *A history of cancer control in the United States with emphasis on the period 1946–1971.* Los Angeles: School of Public health, UCLA.

Breslow, L., & Breslow, N. (1993). Health practices and disability. Some evidence from Alameda County. *Preventive Medicine.*

Breslow, L., Ellis, J., Eaton M., & Kleinman, G. (1951). The California Tumor Registry. *California Medicine, 74,* 179–184.

Breslow, L., & Enstrom, J. (1980). Persistence of health habits and their relationship to mortality. *Preventive Medicine, 9,* 469–483.

Breslow, L., & Goldsmith, J. (1958). Health effects of air pollution. *American Journal of Public Health, 48,* 913–917.

Breslow, L., & Mooney, H. W. (1956). The California morbidity survey. *California Medicine, 84,* 95–97.

Breslow, L., & Ott, N. C. (1954). The California state-wide morbidity survey. *California's Health, 11,* 105–106.

Breslow, L., Shalit, P., & Anderson, G. (1943). Parental and familial factors in the acceptance of diphtheria and smallpox of immunization. *Public Health Reports, 58,* 384–396.

Buechley, R., Drake, R., & Breslow, L. (1958). Height, weight, and mortality in a population of longshoremen. *Journal of Chronic Diseases, 7,* 363–378.

Buell, P., & Breslow, L. (1960). Mortality from coronary heart disease in California men who work long hours. *Journal of Chronic Diseases, 11,* 615–626.

Bureau of Chronic Disease, California State Department of Public Health. (1955). *Clean air for California.* Berkeley, CA: Author.

Burney, L. (1959). Smoking and lung cancer: A statement of the Public Health Service. *Journal of the American Medical Association, 171,* 1829–1837.

California Department of Public Health. (1958). *Health and medical status of Californians.* Berkeley, CA: Author.

California Department of Public Health. (1961). Annual Report.

California Department of Public Health. (1963). *Cigarette smoking and health.* Berkeley, CA: Author.

California Department of Public Health. (1965). Death Records Report CASDPH 1961–1963.

Canelo, G., Bissell, D., Abrams, H., & Breslow, L. (1949). A multiphasic screening survey in San Jose. *California Medicine, 71,* 409–413.

Centers for Disease Control. (1989). *Reducing the health consequences of smoking: 25 years of progress. A report of the Surgeon General.* Department of Health and Human Services, Publication No. (CDC) 89–8411.

Cochrane, A. L. (1972). *Efficiency and effectiveness: Random reflections on health services.* London: Nuffield Hospital Trust.

Collen, M. (Ed.). (1978). *Multiphasic health testing services.* New York: Wiley.

Collins, S. D. (1951). Sickness surveys. In H. Emerson (Ed.), *Administrative medicine* (pp. xx–xx). New York: Nelson and Sons.

Commission on Chronic Illness. (1957a). *Chronic illness in the United States* (Vol. I), *Prevention of chronic illness.* Cambridge, MA: Harvard University Press.

Commission on Chronic Illness. (1957b). *Chronic illness in a large city.* Cambridge, MA: Harvard University Press, The Commonwealth Fund.

Commission on Chronic Illness. (1959). *Chronic illness in a rural area.* Cambridge, MA: Harvard University Press, The Commonwealth Fund.

Committee on the Costs of Medical Care. (1932). *Medical care for the American people: The final report.* Chicago: University of Chicago Press.

Committee on Non-Occupational Health Risks of Asbestiform Fibers, National Research Council. (1984). *Asbestiform fibers: Non-occupational health risks.* Washington, DC: National Academy Press.

Davis, D. (2002). *When smoke ran like water.* New York: Basic Books.

Doll, R., & Hill, A. B. (1952). A study of the etiology of carcinoma of the lung. *British Medical Journal, 2,* 1271–1286.

Drake, R., Buechley, R., & Breslow, L. (1957). An epidemiological investigation of coronary heart disease in the California health survey population. *American Journal of Public Health, 47,* 43–56.

Dublin, L. (1949). *Length of life.* New York: Ronald Free Press.

Evaluation Task Force, California Tobacco Control Program. (2002). *Annual report.* Sacramento, CA: California Department of Health Services, Tobacco Control Section.

Falk, I. (1958, August). The Committee on the Costs of Medical Care—25 years of progress. *American Journal of Public Health.*

Francis, T. (1961). Aspects of the Tecumseh study. *Public Health Reports, 76,* 963.

Glantz. S., Slade, J., Bero, L., Hanauer, P., & Barnes, D. (1996). *The cigarette papers.* Berkeley: University of California Press.

Goldberger, J. (1964). *Goldberger on pellagra.* Baton Rouge: Louisiana State University Press.

Gordon, T., & Kannel, W. B. (1982). Multiple risk factors for predicting coronary heart disease: The concept, accuracy and application. *American Heart Journal, 103,* 1031–1039.

Governor's Advisory Committee on Smoking and Health. (1964). Berkeley, CA: Department of Public Health.

Governor's Committee on Medical Aid and Health. (1960). *Health care for California.* Berkeley: California Department of Public Health.

Haagen-Smit, A. (1963). Photo chemistry and smog. *Journal of the Air Pollution Control Association.*

Halverson, W., Merrill, M., & Breslow, L. (1949). Chronic disease—the chronic disease study of the California Department of Public Health. *American Journal of Public Health, 39,* 593–597.

Hammond, E. C., & Horn, D. (1958). Smoking in relation to death rates. *Journal of the American Medical Association, 166:* 1159–1172, 1294–1308.

Heidbreder, E. (1933). *Seven psychologies.* New York: Appleton-Century-Crofts.

Hochstim, J. R. (1963). *Alternatives to personal interviewing.* Berkeley: California Department of Public Health.

Hochstim, J. R. (1964). *The California Human Population Laboratory for epidemiologic studies.* Berkeley: California Department of Public Health.

Hochstim, J. R. (1967). A critical comparison of three strategies of collecting data from households. *Journal of the American Stat. Association, 629,* 76–89.

Hochstim, J. R. (1970). Health and ways of living—the Alameda County population laboratory. In I. I. Kessler & M. L. Levin (Eds.), *The community as an epidemiologic laboratory.* Baltimore, MD: Johns Hopkins University Press.

Institute of Medicine. (1988). *The future of public health.* Washington, DC: National Academy Press.

Keys, A. (1980). *Seven countries: A multivariate analysis of death and coronary heart disease.* Cambridge, MA: Harvard University Press.

Last, J. (1980). (Ed). *Public health and preventive medicine* (p. 95). Appleton, Century, Crofts.

McGinnis, J. M., & Forge, W. H. (1993). Actual causes of death in the United States. *Journal of the American Medical Association, 270,* 2207–2212.

McKeown, T. (1976). *The role of medicine: Dream, mirage or nemesis.* London: Nuffield Provincial Hospitals Trust.

McKeown, T., & Record, R. G. (1962). Reasons for the decline in mortality in England and Wales during the nineteenth century. *Population Studies, 16,* 94–122.

Morris, J. N., & Crawford, M. D. (1958). Coronary heart disease and physical activity of work. *British Medical Journal, 2,* 1485–1496.

Mullan, F. (2000). Public health then and now. *American Journal of Public Health, 90,* 702–706.

National Cancer Institute Act (1937) Sec. 2.(a).

National Center for Health Statistics, Centers for Disease Control and Prevention. (2003). *Health.* Washington, DC: U.S. Government Printing Office.

National Office of Vital Statistics. (1950). *Vital statistics of the United States* (Vol. 1, p. 209).

Novotny, T., & Siegal, M. (1996). California's tobacco control saga. *Health Affairs,* Spring, 15(1):58–72.

Ochsner, A., & DeBakey, M. (1941). Carcinoma of the lung. *Archives of Surgery, 42,* 209–258.

Paffenbarger, R., Laughlin, M., Gima, A., & Black, R. (1970). Work activity of longshoremen as related to death from coronary heart disease and stroke. *New England Journal of Medicine, 282*(20): 1109–1114.

Pearl, R. (1938). Tobacco smoking and longevity. *Science, 87,* 216–217.

President's Commission on Health Needs of the Nation. (1952). *Building America's health.* Washington, DC: U.S. Government Printing Office.

Renne, K. S. (1974). Measurement of social health on a general population survey. *Social Science Research, 3,* 25–44.

Rosenau, M. (1914). *Preventive medicine and hygiene.* New York: Appleton-Century-Crofts.

Rosenman, R., et al. (1975). Coronary heart disease in the Western Collaborative Group Study: Final follow-up experience of eight and one-half years. *Journal of the American Medical Association, 233,* 872–877.

Sartwell, P. (Ed.). (1965). *Public health and preventive medicine* (9th ed.). New York: Appleton-Century-Crofts.

Sartwell, P. (Ed.). (1973). *Preventive medicine and public health* (10th ed.). New York: Appleton-Century-Crofts.

Selye, H. (1952). *The story of the adaptation syndrome.* Montreal: ACTA.

Sigerist, H. (1943). *Civilization and disease.* Ithaca, NY: Cornell University Press.

Sinai, N., Anderson, O., & Dollar, M. (1946). *Health insurance in the United States.* New York: The Commonwealth Fund.

Surgeon General's Advisory Committee. (1964). *Report on smoking and health.* (PHS Publication No. 1103). Washington, DC: U.S Government Printing Office.

Sydenstriker, E., & Brundage, D. K. (1925). The incidence of illness in a general population group: General results of a morbidity study from December, 1921, through March 31, 1924, in Hagerstown, MD. *Public Health Reports, 40,* 279–291.

Terris, M. (1983). Complex tasks of the second epidemiologic revolution. *Journal of Public Health Policy, 4,* 8–24.

Tobacco Education Oversight Committee. (1993). *Annual report.*

Warner, K. (1985). Cigarette advertising and media coverage of smoking and health. *New England Journal of Medicine, 312,* 384–388.

Webster's Seventh New Collegiate Dictionary. (1963). Springfield, MA: G. and C. Messiam.

World Health Organization. (1948). *World Health Organization charter document.* Geneva, Switzerland: Author.

World Health Organization and UNICEF. (1978). Report of the International Conference on Primary Health Care. Alma-Alta USSR. Geneva: WHO.

World Health Organization—Europe. (1986). *Ottawa charter for health promotion.* Copenhagen, Denmark: Author.

Wynder, E., & Graham, E. (1950). Tobacco smoking as a possible etiologic factor in bronchiogenic carcinoma. *Journal of the American Medical Association, 143,* 329–336.

Index

Springer Publishing Company

Community-Based Health Research
Issues and Methods

Daniel S. Blumenthal, MD, MPH
Ralph J. DiClemente, PhD, Editors

"The editors of this book bring together in one place a description both of epidemiological methods and a discussion of community-level issues. It is a volume that will prove useful to those who wish to conduct contemporary community-based research."

—from the Foreword by **David Satcher,** MD, PhD

This book identifies key concepts of successful community-based research beyond the aspect of location, including prevention focus, population-centered partnerships, multidisciplinary cooperation, and cultural competency. Lessons from the Tuskegee Syphilis Study and case studies on HIV/AIDS prevention and cardiovascular risk reduction illustrate the application of research methods with both positive and negative outcomes.

Contents:

Part I: Issues

- Community-Based Research: An Introduction, *D.S. Blumenthal and E. Yancey*
- Assessing and Applying Community-Based Research, *C. Evans*
- Public Health Ethics and Community-Based Research: Lessons from the Tuskegee Syphilis Study, *B. Jenkins, C. Jones, and D.S. Blumenthal*
- The View from the Community, *A. Cruz, F. Murphy, N. Nyarko, and D.N.Y. Krall*

Part II: Methods

- Study Designs, Surveys, and Descriptive Studies, *N. Asal and L. Beebe*
- Survey Case Study: The Behavioral Risk Factor Surveillance System, *D. Holtzman*
- Qualitative Methods in Community-Based Research, *C. Sterk and K. Elifson*
- HIV/AIDS Prevention: Case Study in Qualitative Research, *K. Elifson and C. Sterk*
- Community Intervention Trials: Theoretical and Methodological Considerations, *R.J. DiClemente, R.A. Crosby, C. Sionean, and D. Holtgrave*
- Cardiovascular Risk Reduction Community Intervention Trials, *S.K. Davis*

2004   240pp   0-8261-2025-3   hard

11 West 42nd Street, New York, NY 10036-8002 • Fax: 212-941-7842
Order Toll-Free: 877-687-7476 • Order On-line: www.springerpub.com

Springer Publishing Company

Introduction to
the U.S. Health Care System
5th Edition

Steven Jonas, MD, MPH, FACPM

"Dr. Jonas has been a voice in the wilderness preaching sense about both health and health services for years. He clearly identifies the problems and issues facing the system and its beneficiaries, based upon the evidence he has carefully marshaled for the reader...and he challenges the reader to make sense out of the facts..."

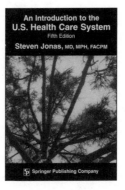

—from the Foreword by **Anthony R. Kovner**, PhD
Professor of Health Policy and Management
New York University, Robert F. Wagner
Graduate School of Public Health

This bestselling text is a concise and balanced classic presenting the domestic health care system. It explains the five major components of the U.S. health care system: health care institutions, health care personnel, financing mechanisms, research and educational institutions that produce biomedical knowledge. Completely updated to reflect the continual changes in the U.S. health care delivery system, this text includes new information on government and public policy reforms and recommendations, as well as website resources and glossary of terms.

Partial Contents:
- An Overview of the US Health Care System
- Institutions: Hospitals
- Institutions: Primary and Ambulatory Care
- Financing and Payment
- Government and the Health Care System
- Health Planning: Principles and Practice
- From Group Medical Practice to Managed Care
- National Health Insurance and National Health Care Reform

2003   234pp   0-8261-3986-8   soft

11 West 42nd Street, New York, NY 10036-8002 • Fax: 212-941-7842
Order Toll-Free: 877-687-7476 • Order On-line: www.springerpub.com